PARESTHESIA

Edited by **Luiz E. Imbelloni**
and **Marildo A. Gouveia**

Paresthesia
Edited by Luiz E. Imbelloni and Marildo A. Gouveia

Published by InTech
Janeza Trdine 9, 51000 Rijeka, Croatia

Publishing Process Manager Adriana Pecar

Technical Editor Teodora Smiljanic

Cover Designer InTech Design Team

Additional hard copies can be obtained from orders@intechopen.com

Paresthesia, Edited by Luiz E. Imbelloni and Marildo A. Gouveia
p. cm.
ISBN 978-953-51-0085-0

For EU product safety concerns:
IN TECH d.o.o., Prolaz Marije Krucifikse Kozulić 3, 51000 Rijeka, Croatia,
info@intechopen.com or visit our website at intechopen.com.

Meet the editors

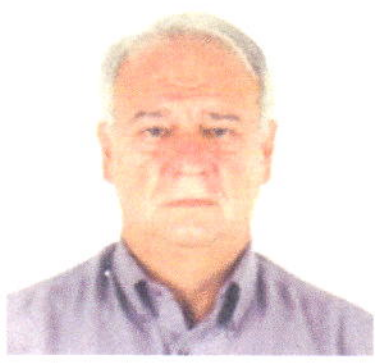

Dr Luiz Eduardo Imbelloni is currently an associate director of the Regional Anesthesia Institute and a Professor at the School of Medicine, Faculdade de Medicina Nova Esperança. He earned the title of Professor Etranger, Universite Louis Pasteur in Strasbourg, France, in 1981. Professor Imbelloni has published extensively in the field of spinal anesthesia and peripheral nerve blocks, and has also authored two books about spinal anesthesia in Brazil. His main research interest is the spinal anesthesia, and he recently published a study on magnetic resonance imaging of the thoracic spine, opening the field to the use of thoracic spinal anesthesia. Professor Imbelloni is a pioneer in the use of spinal anesthesia for laparoscopic cholecystectomy in Brazil and is currently active in clinical trials for spinal anesthesia and peripheral nerve blocks. He also serves as consultant to two major pharmaceutical companies.

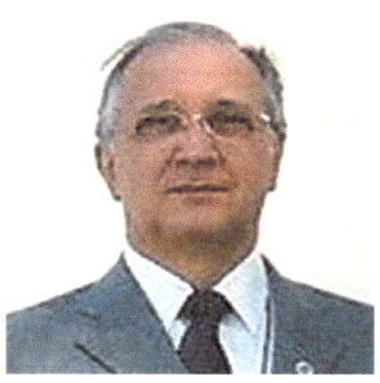

Dr Marildo A. Gouveia was formerly the Head of the Department of Anesthesiology of a State Hospital in the city of Rio de Janeiro. He is now retired of institutional practice and works in private practice in Orthopedics, Plastic Surgery and General Surgery in the city of Rio de Janeiro. He works together with Dr Imbelloni, teaching reginal anesthesia around the continental sized country of Brazil.

Contents

Preface

Paresthesias are spontaneous or evoked abnormal sensations of tingling, burning, pricking, or numbness of a person's skin with no apparent long-term physical effect. Patients generally describe a lancinating or burning pain, often associated with allodynia and hyperalgesia. The manifestation of paresthesia can be transient or chronic. Transient paresthesia can be a symptom of hyperventilation syndrome or a panic attack, and chronic paresthesia can be a result of poor circulation, nerve irritation, neuropathy, or many other conditions and causes.

In older individuals, paresthesia is often the result of poor circulation in the limbs. It can also be a symptom of vitamin deficiency and malnutrition, as well as metabolic disorders like diabetes, hypothyroidism, and hypoparathyroidism, and irritation to the nerve can also come from inflammation of the tissue. Joint conditions, such as rheumatoid or psoriatic arthritis, and carpal tunnel syndrome are also common sources of paresthesia. Another cause of paresthesia, however, can be direct damage to the nerves.

The basic pathophysiology of paresthesias is an altered nerve or nerve pathway function. Paresthesias are thought to represent abnormal showers of impulses generated from an ectopic focus, and can arise from an abnormality anywhere along the sensory pathway, from the peripheral nerves to the sensory cortex. Paresthesias can also be caused by central nervous system or peripheral nervous system abnormalities; central nervous system causes include ischemia, obstruction, compression, infection, inflammation and degenerative conditions. Peripherally induced paresthesias can be caused by entrapment syndromes, metabolic disturbances, trauma, inflammation, connective tissue diseases, toxins, hereditary conditions, malignancies, nutritional deficiencies and other miscellaneous conditions. Confirming the diagnosis and establishing an etiology may require appropriate laboratory and radiologic studies, or possibly other studies as well.

This book is written by authors that are respected in their countries as well as worldwide. Each chapter is written so that everyone can understand, treat and improve the lives of each patient. I hope you will enjoy reading this book.

Dr. Luiz Eduardo Imbelloni
MD, Institute for Regional Anesthesia,
Director of the Institute for Regional Anesthesia,
Hospital de Base-FAMERP, São José do Rio Preto, SP,
Brazil

Dr. Marildo Gouveia
President of LASRA Int'l,
Director of the institute of Regional Anesthesia,
Hospital Mangabeiras, João Pessoa, PB,
Brazil

1

Pathophysiology of Paresthesia

Ibrahim Al Luwimi, Ahmed Ammar and Majed Al Awami
*Department of Neurosurgery and General Surgery,
Cardiothoracic and Vascular Division College of Medicine, University of Dammam,
Kingdom of Saudi Arabia*

1. Introduction

Neuropathic pain arises from a lesion in the somatosensory system, which includes peripheral nerves, spinal dorsal horn, ascending projection tracts, thalamus, the somatosensory cortex and other pain- processing brain region. Patients with neuropathic pain have neurosensory defecits as a consequence of their direct neural injury with positivesensory phenomena (i.e., hyperalgesia, allodyneia, dysthesia and paresthesia). Paresthesia is a variety of neuropathic pain arises as a spontaneous and abnormal sensation. The problem may arise from an abnormality anywhere along the sensory pathway from the peripheral nerves to the sensory cortex. Paresthesia are often described as pins-and-needle sensation. Particular kinds of paresthesias can be seen in the central nervous system (CNS) as follows: focal sensory seizures with cortical lesions, spontaneous pain in the thalamic syndrome, or bursts of paresthesia down the back or into the arms upon flexing the neck (Lhermitte's sign) in patients with multiple sclerosis (MS) or other disorders of the cervical spinal cord. Level lesions of the spinal cord may cause either a band sensation or a girdle sensation, a vague sense of awareness of altered sensation encircling the abdomen. Nerve root lesions or isolated peripheral nerve lesions may also cause paresthesia, but the most intense and annoying paresthesia is due to a multiple symmetric peripheral neuropathy (polyneuropathy). Dysesthesia or allodynia is the term for abnormal sensations ordinarily evoked by a non- noxious stimuli. Paresthesias may be transient (following a prolonged crossing of patients leg) and not associated with neurological abnormality; however, if paresthesias are persistent, sensory system abnormality should be ruled out. In recent years, there has been expanded insight in to the pathophysiology of neuropathic pain because of their multiple and complex pathophysiological mechanisms. Convincing evidence on the relationship between the underlying pathophysiological mechanisms and neuropathic pain symptoms now suggests that classifying neuropathic pain according to a mechanism-based rather than an etiology-based approach. So we will try to explain the mechanism of paresthesia in this chapter.

1.1 Anatomical consideration of sensory transducers

Sensory receptors by means of sensory transduction convert the stimulus from the environment to an action potential for transmission to the brain. The anatomy and classification of these cutaneous sensory nerves has been extensively reviewed by

(Winkelmann, 1988, and Ropper & Samuels, 2009). They are divided in to two groups: the epidermal and the dermal skin-nerve organs. The epidermal skin-nerve organs consist of "free" nerve endings or hederiform nerve organs (e.g., Merkel cells). The term free terminal nerve ending refers to a slight axon expansion that still contains perineural cells including cytoplasm of Schwann cells and multiple cell organelles. In the dermal part, we have free sensory nerve endings, the hair nervous network (Pinkus discs), and the encapsulated endings [Ruffini, Meissner, Krause, Vater-Pacini (vibration), mucocutaneous end organ. Neurophysiological studies have led to a more advanced functional classification of sensory nerves based on the type of cutaneous mechanoreceptor responses. Sensory nerves can be subdivided into four groups: Aα fibers (12–22 mm) are highly myelinated with fast conduction velocity (70–120 m/s), and are associated with muscular spindles and tendon organs. Aß fibers are moderately myelinated (6–12 mm) and capture touch receptors. Aδ fibers constitute a thin myelin sheath (1–5 mm), an intermediate conduction velocity (4–30 m/s), and are generally polymodal. The slow-conducting C fibers (0.5–2m/s) are unmyelinated and small (0.2–1.5 mm). Aδ fibers constitutes almost 80% of primary sensory nerves sprouting from dorsal root ganglia, whereas C fibers make up to almost 20% of the primary afferents. Moreover, the activation threshold of Aδ fibers is higher than that of C fibers. On the molecular level, specific receptor distribution seems to be important for the various functions of sensory nerve subtypes. For example, mechanoreceptors exclusively express the T-type calcium channel Ca (v) 3.2 in the dorsal root ganglion (DRG) of D-hair receptors. Pharmacological blockade indicates that this receptor is important for normal D-hair receptor excitability including mechanosensitivity. However, different mechanisms seem to underlie mechanosensory function in various tissues. The skin is innervated by afferent somatic nerves with fine unmyelinated (C) or myelinated Aδ primary afferent nerve fibers transmitting sensory stimuli (temperature changes, chemicals, inflammatory mediators, pH changes) via dorsal root ganglia and the spinal cord to specific areas of the CNS, resulting in the perception of pain, burning, burning pain, or itching. Thus the skin "talks" to the brain via primary afferents thereby revealing information about the status of peripherally derived pain, pruritus, and local inflammation (Roosterman, et al., 2006).

1.1.1 Normal processing of pain

The study of the complex pathophysiological processes that trigger neuropathic pain comes from animal models of peripheral nerve injuries that was largely designed to mimic human diseases. Several etiological factors were used in these studies such as total nerve transaction or ligation to simulate the clinical conditions of amputation, partial peripheral nerve injury was stimulated by partial nerve ligation. Spinal nerve ligation effectively simulates spinal root damage owing to a lumbar disk herniation. Vincristine, paclitaxel and cisplatin have been used in animal models to mimic polyneuropathy caused by tumor chemotherapy. Finally, experimental model of diabetic neuropathy was produced by induction of damage to pancreatic insulin-producing cells in rats b streptozocin (Leone, et al. 2011). Following peripheral nerve injury, the generation ectopic discharges at the site of stump neuromas due to regenerating sprouts of primary afferent nociceptors has been well documented by microneurography study. There is also formation of abnormal electrical connections between adjacent axons that have been demyelinated. These connections may be responsible for the so-called ephaptic (cross-talk) phenomenon and the crossed after-discharge phenomenon, which occur because the sprouts of primary afferent neurons with damaged peripheral axons can be made to discharge by the discharge of other afferents. Also, locally demyelinated axons can give rise to reflected impulses, which propagate both ortho-and antidromically. This is likely able to produce a dysesthetic buzzing sensation (Sindou, et al. 2001) This process is referred to as peripheral sensitization. The mechanism behind this initially involves the synthesis of arachidonic acid as a result of the action of phospholipase A2 on membrane lipids. Arachidonic acid is then acted upon by cyclo-oxygenase to synthesize prostaglandin that in-turn directly lowers the activation threshold for A-delta and C-fibres.These (Neil, 2011). At the site of injury, inflammatory mediators such as histamine, bradykinin and leukotrienes are released in addition to prostaglandins. These factors are collectively regarded as the 'inflammatory soup' that surrounds peripheral nociceptors resulting in a further reduction in their membrane threshold and activation of dormant receptors. Sensitized receptors display an increased basal (unstimulated) rate of discharge and a supra-normal increase in discharge strength in response to any increase in stimulus. This is easily demonstrated clinically as an area of hyperalgesia extending beyond the boundary of a surgical incision (Neil, 2011). Sodium channel activation underpins the initiation of an action potential and ultimately the perception of acute pain. Following nerve damage, voltage-gated sodium channel expression undergoes marked changes. Abnormal sodium channel Nav1.3, Nav1.7, Nav1.8 and Nav1.9 expression were demonstrated by many studies(Black JA, et al. 2008, Wood JN, et al. 2004, in Leone C, et al. 2011) leading to primary afferent hyperexcitability (a lowered threshold and higher firing rat). The cell body of the sensory afferent fibers lies in the dorsal root ganglia (DRG). Different sodium channels accumulate also within the intact DRG (Amir R 2002, Leone C, et al. 2011). The type III embryonic sodium channel (Nav1.3) might play a key role in the development of neuropathic pain. It is present at low levels in adult afferent nociceptive pathways and after an experimental nerve injury its expression markedly increases (Dib-Hajj, et al. 2009, Leone, et al. 2011). Two human-inherited pain syndromes, inherited erythromelalgia and paroxysmal extreme pain disorder have been linked to the mutations in **SCN9A**, the gene that encodes Nav1.7, whereas loss-of-function mutations in **SCN9A** have been linked to complete insensitivity to pain (Dib-Hajj & Drenth, 2007, Leone, et al., 2011).

1.1.1.1 The role of the cytokines

Proinflammatory cytokines (PICs) such as interleukin-1 β (IL- 1 β), interleukin-6 (IL-6), and tumor necrosis factor- α (TNF α) are an important group of inflammatory mediators and play an essential role in pain sensitization f cytokines. Peripherally, PICs enhance the activity of TRPV1 (transient receptor potential subtype V1) (Nicol et al., 1997; Opree and Kress, 2000; Jin & Gereau, 2006; Kawasaki et al., 2008), induced the expression of pronociceptive genes in dorsal root ganglion (DRG) neurons (Fehrenbacher et al., 2005; von Banchet et al., 2005 in Kawasaki et.al, 2008), and further increase spontaneous activity in DRG neurons (Schafers et al., 2003; Kawasaki et.al, 2008). PICs also enhance pain via central mechanisms. First, PICs are induced in the spinal cord, especially in glial cells (e.g., microglia and astrocytes), in different chronic pain conditions. Second, intrathecal injection of the PICs was shown to enhance pain. Third, spinal blockade of PIC signaling attenuates chronic pain. The study of Kawasaki et al., 2008, have demonstrated that PICs induce central sensitization and hyperalgesia via distinct and overlapping synaptic mechanisms in superficial dorsal horn neurons either by increasing excitatory synaptic transmission or by decreasing inhibitory synaptic transmission. PICs may further induce long-term synaptic plasticity through cAMP response element-binding protein (CREB)-mediated gene transcription. Blockade of PIC signaling could be an effective way to suppress central sensitization and alleviate chronic pain. Various protein regulation is seen in peripheral sensitization, peripheral nerve injury induced by various animal studies changes transient receptor potential (TRP) channel expression. TRP channels are a family of nonselective cation-permeable channels that are known to be important for sensory signaling in the peripheral nervous system. Vanilloid receptor 1 (TRPV1), a member of the TRP family, was investigated for their role in the development of neuropathic pain. Total or partial sciatic nerve transection, or spinal nerve ligation, reduce TRPV1 expression in the somata of all damaged dorsal root ganglia. Following partial nerve lesion or spinal nerve ligation, TRPV1 expression is greater in the undamaged dorsal root ganglion somata than in controls. TRPV1-deficient mice lack hyperalgesia and TRPV1 antagonists reduce pain behavior in mice after spinal nerve ligation. This is a strong evidence that TRPV1 plays a crucial role in the development of neuropathic pain (Staaf et al., 2009, Hudson, et al. 2001, Baron & Caterina, et al., 2000, Leone et al., 2011). The physiological changes seen within inflamed or infected tissue (i.e. heat and acidic pH) are known to activate the TPRV-1 receptor and enhance pain sensitivity. Other molecules within nociceptors that are known to enhance pain transmission include substance-P and calcitonin gene related peptide (CGRP). These two factors are often released simultaneously within the cell. Substance P activates second order neurons that send a 'pain' signal to the brain while CGRP contributes to neurogenic inflammation by causing vasodilation and hence warmth, redness and swelling (Neil, 2011). Normally, the DRG cell body receives via the nerve terminal signal substances, which modify gene transcription and protein synthesis. After nerve damage, these molecules will be lost. So, nerve damage, through complex signaling mechanisms (cAMP-dependent PKA and Ca2+/phospholipid-dependent PKC) modulate gene transcription. Also, it was demonstrated by animal study that after nerve damage, there is an induction of c-jun, p-38 and ERK. The encoded proteins of these genes are involved in the inflammatory responses, neuronal degeneration and neuronal plasticity, which maintain pain sensation. Therefore, the importance of genetic factors in neuropathic pain remains an interesting question for further research, especially for their possible use as targets for new, more selective drugs (Hudmon et al., 2008, Stamboulian et al., 2010, Leon , et al., 2011).

1.1.1.2 Central sensitization

The cell bodies of the peripheral afferent pain fibers of both A- δ and C types are placed in the dorsal root ganglia; central extensions of these nerve cells project via the dorsal root to the dorsal horn of the spinal cord (or, in the case of cranial pain afferents, to the nucleus of the trigeminal nerve, the medullary analogue of the dorsal horn). The pain afferents occupy mainly the lateral part of the root entry zone. Within the spinal cord, many of the thinnest fibers (C fibers) form a discrete bundle, the tract of Lissauer (Ropper & Samuels, 2009).

1.1.1.3 The dorsal horn

The afferent pain fibers, after traversing the tract of Lissauer, terminate in the posterior gray matter or dorsal horn, predominantly in the marginal zone. Most of the fibers terminate within the segment of their entry into the cord; some extend ipsilaterally to one or two adjacent rostral and caudal segments; and some project via the anterior commissure to the contralateral dorsal horn. Second-order neurons, the sites of synapse of afferent sensory fibers in the dorsal horn, are arranged in a series of six layers known as Rexed's laminae (Fig.1). Rexed's laminae I, II, and V play a role in modulating nociceptive transmission. A-δ fibers terminate principally in lamina I of Rexed (marginal cell layer of Waldeyer) and also in the outermost part of lamina II; some A- δ pain fibers penetrate the dorsal gray matter and terminate in the lateral part of lamina V . Unmyelinated (C) fibers terminate in lamina II (substantia gelatinosa). Yet other cells that respond to painful cutaneous stimulation are located in ventral horn laminae VII and VIII. The latter neurons are responsive to descending impulses from brainstem nuclei as well as segmental sensory impulses. From` these cells of termination, second-order axons connect with ventral and lateral horn cells in the same and adjacent spinal segments and subserve both somatic and autonomic reflexes. The main bundle of secondary neurons subserving pain sensation projects contralaterally (and to a lesser extent ipsilaterally) to higher levels; this constitutes the spinothalamic tract. Most of the spinothalamic neurons ultimately ascend to the ventroposterolateral nucleus of the thalamus, though they may branch to provide input to these brain stem targets. However, some axons terminate solely in these bulbar regions, which then send projections to thalamic nuclei (Ropper & Samuels, 2009).

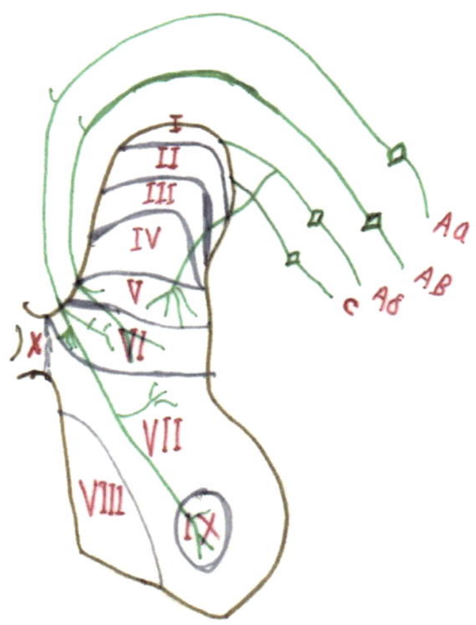

Fig. 1. Diagramatic representation of Rexed's laminae.

Information about this pathway in humans has been derived from the study of postmortem material and from the examination of patients subjected to anterolateral cordotomy for intractable pain. The clinical relevance is seen with the unilateral section of the anterolateral funiculus, which produces a relatively complete loss of pain and thermal sense on the opposite side of the body, extending to a level two or three segments below the lesion as noted earlier. Usually, the pain sensibility returns after a variable period of time, probably being conducted by pathways that lie outside the anterolateral quadrants of the spinal cord that gradually increases their capacity to conduct pain impulses. One of these is a longitudinal polysynaptic bundle of small myelinated fibers in the center of the dorsal horn (the dorsal intracornual tract); another consists of axons of lamina I cells that travel in the dorsal part of the lateral funiculus (Ropper & Samuels, 2009). The second-order nociceptive neurons consist of nociceptive-specific neurons and wide dynamic range neurons (Craig,

2006, D'Mello, 2008, Leone, et al., 2011). Nociceptive-specific neurons are located in the outer layers (laminae I–II) of the dorsal horn; wide dynamic range neurons lie in deeper laminae (most of lamina V neurons are wide dynamic neurons). Nociceptive-specific neurons respond selectively to noxious stimuli conveyed by Aδ- and C-fibers. Wide dynamic range neurons excited both by noxious and non-noxious stimuli, receive both large-myelinated Aβ-fibers as well as Aδ- and C-fibers. Wide dynamic range neurons can encode and project different types of sensory information, nociceptive and non-nociceptive, varying their firing rate (higher for noxious and lower for non-noxious stimuli).

Nociceptive neurons usually have a localized receptive field and probably plays an important role in spatially detecting nociceptive stimuli. By contrast, wide dynamic range neurons have a large receptive field and a stimulus-response function (the higher the stimulus intensity, the higher the firing rate of their output), their main function is to detect and discriminate the intensity of noxious stimuli (Dubner 1985, Sessle 1991, Leone, et al., 2011). The fundamental process of central sensitization is the release of the primary afferent neuron that binds to the NMDA receptor resulting in an influx of calcium and potassium. This leads to nerve depolarization and heightened sensitivity to circulating neurotransmitter. The N-methyl, D-adenine (NMDA) receptor is found widely within the CNS but features prominently in the DRG. At the molecular level, nociception induces alteration in second order neurone such as phosphorylation of NMDA and AMPA receptors. These processes contribute to the process of central sensitization (Neil, 2011). At the dorsal horn usually two processes occur, which are designated "windup" and "central sensitization. Central sensitization has been described earlier, the "windup" results from repetitive C-fiber firing at low frequencies that results in a progressive buildup of the amplitude of the response of the dorsal horn neuron, only during the repetitive train. Both can be blocked by NMDA receptor antagonists. Central sensitization can result from windup. This is a result of the calcium influx through the NMDA receptor following depolarization of the dorsal horn membrane. The intracellular calcium activates a number of kinase among which protein kinase C (PKC) is likely important. PKC enhances the NMDA receptor, which results in subsequent glutamate binding of the NMDA receptor generating an inward current. Though windup can result in central sensitization, it is not necessary for central sensitization to occur (Brannagan,2010). The neurotransmitters on activiation of NMDA receptor-channel produce an increase of intracellular Ca2+ and cAMP concentrations, which activates protein kinase. Protein kinase consist of the signaling cascade that modulates gene transcription (i.e. c-fos, c-jun) (Ji et al., 2003, Willis et al., 2002, Leone et al., 2011).

1.1.1.4 Role of calcium currents in the genesis of neuropathic pain

Cytoplasmic Ca2+ regulates numerous cellular processes in neurons. The pathogenic contribution of altered inward Ca2+ flux (ICa) through voltage gated Ca2+ channels in sensory neurons after peripheral nerve injury was examine by Hogan (2007). Primary sensory neurons isolated from animals after peripheral nerve injury with partial ligation show a decrease in high-voltage activated ICa by approximately one third. Low voltage-activated ICa is nearly eliminated by peripheral nerve injury. Loss of ICa leads to decreased activation of Ca2+-activated K+ currents, which are also directly reduced in traumatized neurons. As a result of these changes in membrane currents, membrane voltage recordings show increased action potential duration and diminished after hyperpolarization.

Excitability is elevated, as indicated by resting membrane potential depolarization and a decreased current threshold for action potential initiation. Traumatized nociceptive neurons develop increased repetitive firing during sustained depolarization after axotomy. Concurrently, cytoplasmic Ca2+ transients are diminished. In conclusions, axotomized neurons, especially pain-conducting ones, develop instability and elevated excitability after peripheral injury. DRG neurons expressed a variety of voltage-gated Ca2+ channels (VGCCs). High voltage activated (HVA) are distinguished by their voltage dependency, kinetics, and pharmacology. Low voltage activated (LVA) currents, or T currents inactivate rapidly during sustained depolarization but close (deactivate) slowly after repolarization of the membrane. Because of these features, T-currents account for up to 50% of Ca2+ entry. DRG neurons show definite heterogeneity with respect to HVA Ca2+ channels. Nerve injury, particularly axotomy, results in a loss of ICa in primary sensory neurons, which is present after different types of injury and their role in generating neuropathic pain. Axotomized Aδ neurons develop increased repetitive firing during sustained depolarization after axotomy , whereas Aα/β neurons does not. Thus, axotomized neurons, especially pain-conducting ones, develop instability and elevated excitability. Altered function of other ionic membrane channels contributes to the disordered membrane biophysics observed after nerve injury, including substantial changes in voltage-gated Na+ and K+ channels (Hogan, 2007).

1.1.1.5 The role of glial cells in neuropathic pain

Glial cells, including microglia and astrocytes, are non-neuronal cells that have various functions in the spinal cord. They act as physical support, release mediators that modulate neuronal activity and alter axonal and dendritic growth. Usually they account for 70% of CNS cells under normal conditions. Uncontrolled glial cell activation under neuropathic pain conditions induces the release of proinflammatory cytokines and other substances that facilitate pain transmission (Watkins 2009, Mika 2008, Song 2001, Leone et al., 2011). In addition, glial cells enhance release of substance P and excitatory amino acids from nerve terminals, including primary afferents in the spinal cord (Malcangio 1996, Inoue 1999, Leone, et al., 2011). Their activation can also lead to altered opioid system activity (Watkins 2009, Mika 2008, Song 2001, Leone et al., 2011). Neuropathic pain can also induce a protein named fractalkine, which is expressed by neuron (Abbadie 2009, Leone et al., 2011). The soluble portion of fractalkine diffuses away and binds to and activates glial cells (Chapman 2000, Leone et al., 2011). Intrathecal fractalkine creates both thermal hyperalgesia and mechanical allodynia, and fractalkine receptor blockade blocks inflammatory neuropathy-induced pain (Milligan, 2004, Leone et al., 2011).

1.1.1.6 Thalamic projection of pain fibers

The lateral division of the spinothalamic tract terminates in the ventrobasal and posterior groups of nuclei, the most important of which is the VPL nucleus. The medial portion terminates mainly in the intralaminar complex of nuclei and in the nucleus submedius. Spinoreticulothalamic (paleospinothalamic) fibers project onto the medial intralaminar (primarily parafascicular and centrolateral) thalamic nuclei. Projections from the dorsal column nuclei, which have a modulating influence on pain transmission, are mainly terminated in the ventrobasal and ventroposterior group of nuclei (Ropper & Samuels, 2009).

1.1.1.7 Thalamocortical projections

The ventrobasal thalamic complex and the ventroposterior group of nuclei project to two main cortical areas: the primary sensory (postcentral) cortex (a small number terminate in the precentral cortex) and the upper bank of the Sylvian fissure. They are concerned mainly with the reception of tactile and proprioceptive stimuli and with all discriminative sensory functions including pain (Ropper & Samuels, 2009).

1.1.1.8 Descending pain-modulating systems

The descending fibers play an important role to modulate activity in nociceptive pathways and inhibition of neuropathic pain. The endogenous pain control system decend from the frontal cortex and hypothalamus and projects to cells in the peri-aqueductal region of the midbrain and then passes to the ventromedial medulla. From there it descends in the dorsal part of the lateral fasciculus of the spinal cord to the posterior horns (laminae I, II, and V). Several other descending pathways, noradrenergic and serotonergic, arise in the locus ceruleus, dorsal raphe nucleus, and nucleus reticularis. Gigantocellularis are also important modifiers of the nociceptive response. The descending pain-control systems mainly acting via noradrenergic and serotonergic, as well as opiate pathway. A descending norepinephrine- pathway, also has been traced from the locus ceruleus in the dorsolateral pons to the spinal cord, and its activation blocks spinal nociceptive neurons. The rostroventral medulla contains a large number of serotonergic neurons from which descending fibers inhibit dorsal horn cells concerned with pain transmission, this provide a rationale for the use of serotonin agonists antidepression medications in patients with chronic pain (Ropper & Samuels, 2009).

1.1.1.9 Genetic inheritance of neuropathic pain

Genetic risk factors play as an important factor in various clinical neuropathic pain conditions. Various genetic diseases are reported to be associated with an increased risk for the development of neuropathic pain. For example, Fabry disease, which is a rare X-linked recessive (inherited) lysosomal storage disease that causes painful neuropathy (Zarate et al., 2008, Leone, et al., 2011). Mutations in SCN9A, the gene that encodes Nav1.7 caused two extremely rare inherited neuropathic pain conditions, erythromelalgia and paroxysmal extreme pain disorder (Dib-Hajj et al., 2007, Leone et al., 2011). Following nervous system damage, gene mutations can lead to the genetic risk of developing neuropathic pain. To highlight the role of genetic susceptibility in neuropathic pain, a recent study investigates a single nucleotide polymorphism association of the potassium channel α subunit, KCNS1, in humans with neuropathic pain. They found that a common amino acid changing-allele, the 'valine risk allele', was significantly associated with higher pain scores (Costigan et al., 2010, Leone et al., 2011). Other studies investigated catechol-O-methyltransferase polymorphisms that modulate nociceptive and dysfunctional temporomandibular joint disorder pain (Diatchenko et al., 2005, Nackley et al., 2006, Leone et al., 2011). A single nucleotide polymorphism in SCN9A is demonstrated by recent study to increase the firing frequency of DRG neurons, another study demonstrates that this single nucleotide polymorphism was subsequently shown to be associated with chronic pain (Reimann et al., 2010, Estacion et al., Leone et al. 2011). So, a new future approach to neuropathic pain should include genetic analysis among the more conventional diagnostic tools.

1.1.2 Pathophysiologic characteristic of paresthesia

Human microneurography experiments have demonstrated that tingling paresthesia results from the aberrant activity of mechanosensitive neurons (Ochoa and Torebjork 1980, Nordin et al., 1984, Lennertz et al., 2010), but little is known about the molecular mechanisms underlying this abnormal sensation. So Hydroxy-sanshool (sanshool), which is a natural plant alkylamide that induces numbing and robust tingling paresthesia in humans (Bryant and Mezine, 1999; Sugai et al., 2005, in Lennertz, et al., 2010) has been used to provide insight into the cellular and molecular mechanisms underlying tingling paresthesia. Nearly 52% of cultured dorsal root ganglion neurons are excited by sanshool in vitro, including a: subset of large-diameter, putative light-touch mechanoreceptors (Bautista et al., 2008, Lennertz, et al., 2010)). Lingual nerve (Bryant and Mezine, 1999 , Lennertz, et al., 2010) and dorsal horn neurons recording (Sawyer et al., 2009, Lennertz, et al., 2010) confirm that sanshool does activate light-touch receptors. Interestingly, it was found that sanshool may discriminate between subtypes of mechanosensitive fibers. Using the saphenous skin–nerve preparation to record from primary afferent nerve fibers ex vivo, it was demonstrated that sanshool excites specific subtypes of cutaneous mechanoreceptors. Sanshool potently activates all ultrasensitive D-hair fibers and, to a lesser extent, unique populations of pressure-sensitive Aß fibers and low conduction velocity C fibers. In all fiber types, sanshool evokes action potential bursting, reminiscent of the activity observed in myelinated fibers of human subjects experiencing tingling paresthesia. In addition, sanshool-evoked avoidance behavior is distinct from pain-evoked behaviors and is consistent with the robust activation of low threshold mechanoreceptors. Moreover, it was proved that sanshool is an invaluable tool for delineating the function of novel mechanosensitive neuron subtypes (Lennertz et al., 2010). Thus, the majority of fibers activated by sanshool are Aβ and D-hair neurons that mediate the detection of light-touch rather than noxious stimuli. However, there is a subset of C fibers that do respond robustly to sanshool. In a subset of fibers, sanshool evoked a burst pattern of action potential firing. Bursting was most prevalent among sanshool-sensitive C fibers and D-hair fibers, occurring in 73 and 26% of sanshool-sensitive fibers, respectively. Large myelinated Aβ fibers were the least likely to show bursting because only one RA- Aβ fiber exhibited bursting and none of the SA- Aβ fibers displayed bursting Interestingly, the rapidly adapting D-hair fibers and slowly adapting C fibers displayed distinct patterns of burst firing. Rapidly adapting D-hair fibers (and the RA- Aβ fiber) issued quick bursts of action potentials with short intervals, whereas the slowly adapting C fibers issued significantly longer duration bursts of action potentials at less frequent intevals. Consequently, the average number of action potentials per burst was considerably higher in C fibers than in D-hair or RA- Aβ fibers. Sanshool is the first pharmacological agent identified that can discriminate between subsets of mechanosensory neurons which often leads to tingling paresthesia in patients . Among Aδ fibers, virtually all D-hair afferents were vigorously excited by sanshool, whereas adrenomedullin (AM) nociceptors were completely unresponsive. D-hair afferents are the most sensitive of all mechanoreceptors, with mechanical thresholds below the measurable limit D-hairs have also been implicated in diabetic peripheral neuropathy (Shin et al., 2003; Jagodic et al., 2007, Lennerts et al., 2010), which often leads to tingling paresthesia in patients(Lennertz et al., 2010).

Sanshool activates rapidly adapting mylinated more better than slowly adapting fibers. Spontaneous activity in rapidly adapting myelinated fibers has been implicated in both injury- and disease-evoked paresthesia, as well as in post ischemic paresthesia; however, the exact neuronal subtypes that mediate tingling paresthesia have not been characterized (Ochoa and Torebjrko, 1980; Nordin et al., 1984, Lennertz, et al., 2010). A subset of slowly adapting Aβ fibers also responded to sanshool, two findings support the idea that the sanshool-sensitive slowly adapting Aβ fibers are SA-II type skin stretch sensors. First, the proportion of sanshool-sensitive slowly adapting Aβ fibers (36%) is consistent with the proportion of SA-II type skin stretch sensors. Second, the sanshool-sensitive SA- Aβ fibers were approximately fivefold less sensitive to sustained force than the sanshool-insensitive population. Sanshool activated a unique subset of C fibers that has an intrinsically slower conduction velocity than other C fibers (Lennertz et al., 2010). Previous studies of tingling paresthesia in humans have failed to report aberrant activity of Aδ or C fibers (Ochoa and Torebjork, 1980; Nordin et al., 1984, Lennertz, et al., 2010). However, this may be attributable to technical difficulties in recording from patients experiencing tingling paresthesia. Knowing that sanshool elicits tingling paresthesia through selective activation of mechanosensitive somatosensory neurons. Also, sanshool consumption fails to elicit the nocifensive responses of nose rubbing and wiping that are commonly observed after consumption of capsaicin or mustard oil (our unpublished observations)(Lennertz et al., 2010).Thus, sanshool evoked behaviors is more likely to be resulted from tingling paresthesia rather than painful irritation and this is consistent with the activation pattern of Aδ and Aβ fibers by sanshool, as well as with results from human psychophysical studies demonstrating that sanshool does not elicit pain sensations (Bryant and Mezine, 1999; Sugai et al., 2005, Lennertz et al., 2010). Although sanshool also activates a subset of C fibers, it is unclear whether these C fibers actually transmit pain signals. Several studies have demonstrated the existence of C fibers that transmit information other than pain, such as the study by (Loken et al., 2009, Lennertz, et al., 2010), who demonstrates the existence of unmyelinated C fibers that code for pleasant touch sensations in humans. In addition, C fibers that transmit sensations of brushing and itch have also been reported (Zotterman, 1939, Lennertz, et al., 2010). Specific labeling of neurons that express a mass-related G-protein-coupled receptor, MrgprB4, revealed a unique subpopulation of C fibers that specifically innervate the skin but not the viscera. These fibers are hypothesized to function as touch receptors rather than nociceptors (Liu et al., 2007, Lennertz, et al., 2010). Common among all subtypes of sanshool-sensitive fibers is the presence of action potential bursting, which we observed in 29% of fibers. Bursting is also associated with tingling paresthesia. Microelectrode recordings show robust bursting of sensory afferents in normal human subjects experiencing tingling paresthesia (Ochoa and Torebjork, 1980, Lennertz et al., 2010). Neuronal recordings from patients suffering from activity-dependent tingling paresthesia showed that robust bursting of myelinated, rapidly adapting mechanoreceptors increased with the degree of paresthesia. Also, it was found in a rat models of diabetic neuropathy, robust bursting of medium-diameter fibers increased in diabetic neurons compared with wild-type neurons (Jagodic et al., 2007, Lennertz, et al., 2010). Bursting is exhibited by many neurons within the CNS, as well as some peripheral neurons. In the peripheral nervous system, bursting has been described in trigeminal afferents in the brainstem that are thought to play a key role in the central pattern generator circuit regulating mastication in rodents (Brocard et al., 2006; Hsiao et al., 2009, Lennertz, et al., 2010). In addition, neuronal recordings from patients suffering from activity-dependent tingling paresthesia showed robust bursting of myelinated, rapidly adapting mechanoreceptors that increased with the degree of paresthesia. Finally, in rat models of diabetic neuropathy, robust bursting of medium-diameter fibers increased in diabetic neurons compared with wild-type neurons (Jagodic et al., 2007, Lennertz, et al., 2010). It has been demonstrated that sanshool-evoked fiber responses are of similar prevalence and amplitude in the presence or absence of TRPA1 and TRPV1 selective antagonists. These data suggest that neither TRPA1 nor TRPV1 mediate the excitatory effects of sanshool (Lennertz et al., 2010). Sanshool may act directly on two pore potassium channel (KCNK) in sensory neurons as well as in keratinocytes, which are known to modulate sensory neuron function (Koizumi et al., 2004; Lumpkin and Caterina, 2007; Lennertz et al., 2010) to induce tingling paresthesia, and that is because in somatosensory neurons, expression and electrophysiological studies show the presence of KCNK18 channels (Dobler et al., 2007; Kang et al., 2008, Lennertz et al., 2010), and expression of KCNK3 and KCNK9 have not been demonstrated. However, KCNK3 and KCNK9 are expressed by keratinocytes in the skin (Kang and Kim, 2006, Lennertz, et al., 2010). Bursting in trigeminal neurons has been linked to the activity of Kv1 channels (Hsiao et al., 2009). Characterization of sanshool-sensitive mechanoreceptors represents an essential first step in identifying the cellular and molecular mechanisms underlying tingling paresthesia that accompanies peripheral neuropathy and injury (Lennertz, et al., 2010).

1.1.3 Paresthesia and entrapment neuropathy

Paresthesia are reported in many different conditions of entrapment neuropathies (Lewis, 2010). In our study of surgical outcome of thoracic outlet compression syndrome, paresthesia was the second most common syndrome (30%) after pain (86.7%), two-thirds of the patient were operated (Al Luwimi &Al Awami, 2009). Recently symptoms of paresthesia and signs of numbness were recorded by (Hann et al., 2010) to establish the changes in nerve excitability and symptom generation associated with the application of focal nerve compression (FNC). The aim of the study was to investigate the changes in sensory nerve excitability and thereby resting membrane potential that develops with focal nerve compression (FNC). FNC was applied by means of a custom-designed, novel compression device (Fig 2).

Paraesthesia developed in response to application of FNC. Their intensity increased as the FNC continued reaching the end of FNC (Fig. 3A). Following the release of FNC, paraesthesia continued and the duration required for complete resolution of symptoms varied between individuals, ranging from 3 to 11 min. Numbness was quantitatively assessed using von frey filaments(VFFs). The levels of numbness, as indicated by normalized VFFs, paralleled the pattern of changes produced by paraesthesiae (Fig. 3B). During FNC, the mean tactile sensitivity deteriorated, followed by a gradual recovery with release of FNC.

1.1.3.1 Comparison to ischaemia

The ischemia change seen on release of compression was similar to that previously achieved with generalized limb ischaemia (Fig. 4A), similarly, the reduction in compound sensory action potential (CSAP) amplitude observed during compression was similar to that achieved with ischaemia (Fig. 4B), suggesting that the two maneuvres achieved comparable effects on the axons over similar time period. But, the rates of recovery on release of the different interventions were clearly different, the rate of compound sensory action potential

(CSAP) recovery was significantly faster following release of FNC (12.4 +/- 2.1% min−1) when compared to ischaemia (3.6 +/- 0.6% min−1; P <0.005). Accordingly, full recovery of CSAP was achieved in a shorter time frame with release of FNC (3.3 +/- 0.5min) than ischaemia (8.8 +/- 2.1min; P <0.05(Hann, et al., 2010).

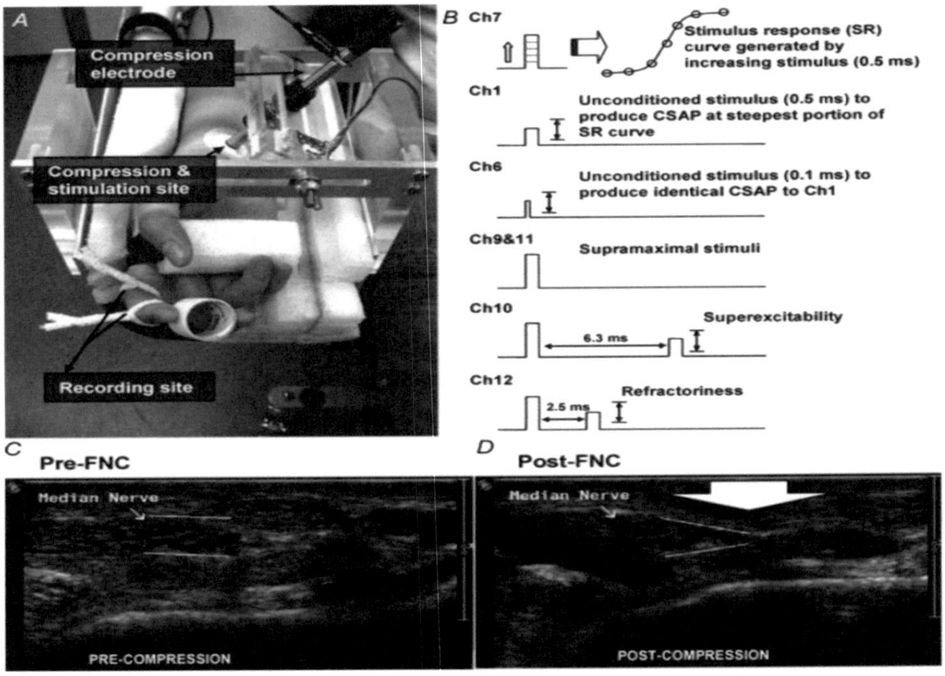

Fig. 2. Experimental paradigm and structural changes to the median nerve achieved via FNC. **A**, experimental protocol. The median nerve was stimulated at the wrist and the resultant compound sensory action potential (CSAP) was recorded from the second digit. A custom designed and built compression device was utilized for delivering both electrical stimulation and focal nerve compression. **B**, configuration of stimulation channels. Vertical arrows in channels 1, 6, 10 and 12 indicate threshold tracking of the test stimulus, aiming to generate a CSAP amplitude corresponding to the steepest portion of SR curve in channel 7. **C**, a representative cross-sectional ultrasound (US) image of median nerve (MN) prior to FNC. **D**, cross-sectional US image of MN immediately after the application of FNC showing the changes in shape of MN. Open vertical arrow indicates the region of FNC application. Copy permission from publisher (John Wiley and Sons) via Copyright Clearance Center's Rights Link service from the article by Hann S.E, J Physiol 588.10 (2010) pp 1737–1745.

When paraesthesia generation was compared between the process of FNC and ischemia it was continued to increase during the former process of FNC, and subsided after initial changes during the latter process (Fig. 3C) (Han et al., 2008, 2010). On the release of FNC, there was no increase in paraesthesia, in contrast with the release of ischaemia (of similar duration), where a large rebound in the intensity of paraesthesia developed. The pattern of change for numbness during and after FNC was similar to that observed with an ischaemic insult (Fig. 3D) (Han et al., 2008, 2010). There appeared apparent relationship between the pattern of paraesthesia and corresponding changes in strength–duration time constant (SDTC). The pattern of paraesthesia generation observed in the present series was novel (Fig. 3A and C). The metabolic changes seen in the process of ischemia and FNC are different and that might explain the change in paresthesia generation in the two processes. The metabolic byproducts of ischaemia, such as H+, which accumulate and potentially interfere with parameters that determine axonal excitability, particularly the Na+/K+-ATPase and persistent Na+ conductance's. H+ ions and pH can modify channel gating (Wanke et al., 1980, 1983, Hann, et al. 2010), raised intracellular pH reduce Na+ channel inactivation (Brodwick & Eaton, 1978, Hann et al., 2010). Also, low pH may also alter the gating mode of persistent Na+ conductances (Baker & Bostock, 1999; Hann et al., 2010).

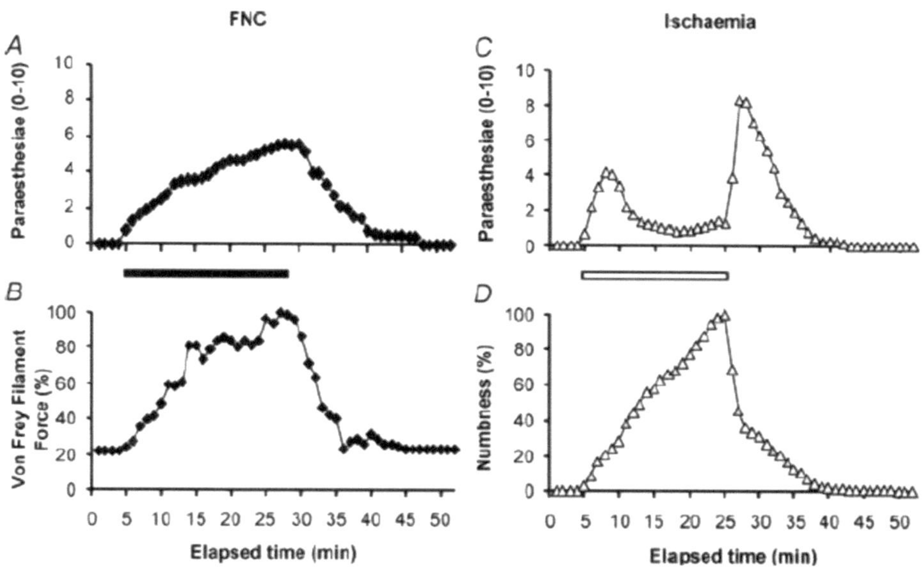

Fig. 3. Symptom rating before, during and after FNC (A and B), and compared to ischaemia (C and D). Copy permission from publisher (John Wiley and Sons) via Copyright Clearance Center's RightsLink service from the article by Hann S.E, J Physiol 588.10 (2010) pp 1737–1745.

Both processes can contribute to greater rate of paraesthesia generation during the initial phases of generalized ischaemia compared to FNC (Fig. 3A and C). But, during FNC where focal ischaemia appeared to be the underlying mechanism, metabolites exerted less significant effects. Such a view would also be supported by the rapid rate of CSAP recovery observed with release of FNC. Such differences in the secondary effects on axonal function, and persistent Na+ conductances, may also contribute to the relative differences in (SDTC) and symptom generation observed between FNC and ischaemia, particularly the relative absence of paraesthesia on release of FNC, in contrast to the more severe symptoms that follow generalized ischaemia (Fig. 5A). It is possible that metabolites associated with generalized ischaemia enhanced the accumulation of K+ ions during ischaemic depolarization, and it is possible that this mechanism dose not contribute in the process of FNC. So, Post-ischaemic paraesthesia is most likely due to regenerative potassium currents (Han et al.; Kuwabara, 2008; Hann et al., 2010). In addition, different mechanisms were described for the peak of paraesthesia during and after ischaemia, (Kuwabara, 2008). During ischaemia, paraesthesia appear to be of low frequency ('buzzing'), and have been attributed to persistent Na+ conductances (Kiernan & Bostock, 2000; Han et al., 2008, 2009, 2010). In the post-ischaemic period, the discharges are typically of high frequency, occurring in recurrent bursts, attributed to inward K+ currents. The origin of such activity appears to be rapidly adapting or Meissner's corpuscle mechanoreceptor fibres (Ochoa & Torebjork, 1980; Kuwabara, 2008; Hann et al., 2010). Additional modifying factors including stretch sensitive channels (Hamill, 2006; Hann et al., 2010) and morphological changes involving the axonal membrane (Clarke et al., 2007; Hann et al., 2010) cannot be excluded.

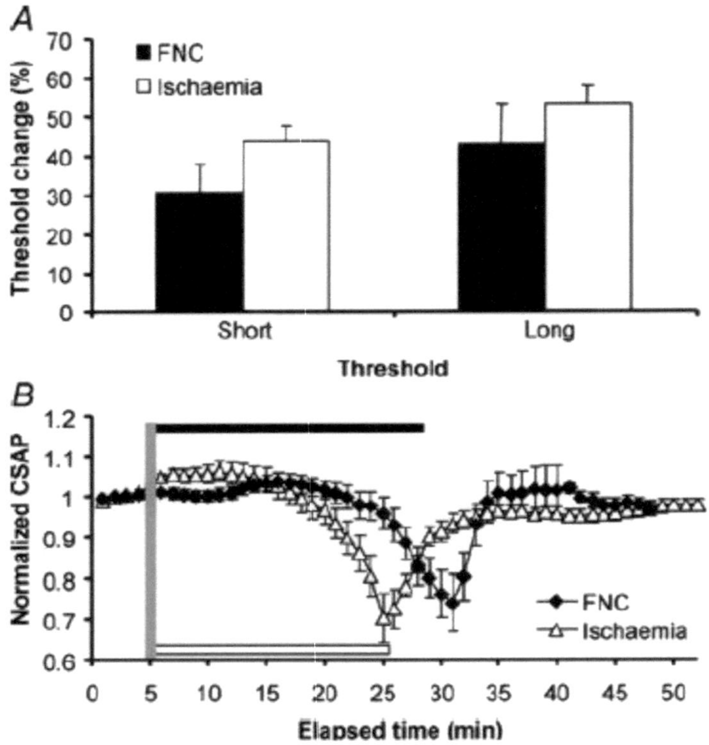

Fig. 4. Comparison between FNC applied to the wrist and ischaemia applied to the upper limb for associated threshold and supramaximal response. **A**, the maximal threshold change achieved following release of compression and ischaemia. **B**, normalized compound sensory action potential(CSAP) amplitude, with similar reductions achieved for both FNC (filled diamonds) and ischaemia (open diamonds). Horizontal bar indicates period of FNC (filled) or ischaemia (open), and grey vertical bar represents the period to achieve compression. Copy permission from publisher (John Wiley and Sons) via Copyright Clearance Center's RightsLink service from the article by Hann S.E, J Physiol 588.10 (2010) pp 1737-1745.

1.1.4 Mechanisms of paresthesia in dental procedures

The mechanism of paresthesia in dental procedure depend on the pharmacology of the dental local anesthetics and their local action. These local anesthetics are classified into esters and amides based on the bond hydrolyzed in metabolic degradation and elimination in the human body (Ritchie & Greene, 1985; Nickel, 1990). The hydrolysis of the ester or amide bond, which is joining the three parts of the local anesthetics molecule, the aromatic (hydrophobic), the alcoholic (hydrophilic) and tertiary amino groups, will results in the formation of an alcohol product which varies in structure and activity depending on the parent molecule (Morrison & Boyed, 1987; Nickel, 1990). This product is an active one, it will increase the length of the alcohol group and thus a greater anesthetic potency. The increase anesthetic potency of the alcohol group because of alcohol is neurotoxic, causing paresthesia (Littler, 1984; Shannon & Wiscott, 1974; Nickel, 1990).

1.1.5 Mechanisms of paresthesias arising from healthy axons

Paresthesia have been described to arise from healthy axons. Cutaneous afferents due to differences in their biophysical properties are more excitable than motor axons, such differences include more persistent Na (+) conductance which create a greater tendency to ectopic activity. These ectopic discharges have been described in normal afferents by different mechanisms such as hyperventilation, ischemia, release of ischemia, and prolonged tetanization. The alkaline shift produced by hyperventilation selectively increases the persistent Na (+) conductance, while the membrane depolarization produced by ischemia affects both transient and persistent Na (+) channels. Post-ischemic and post-tetanic paresthesia occur when hyperpolarization by the Na (+)/K (+) pump is transiently prevented by raised extracellular K (+). The electrochemical gradient for K (+) is reversed, and inward K(+) currents trigger regenerative depolarization. These mechanisms of paresthesia generation can account for paresthesia in normal subjects and may be relevant in some peripheral nerve disorders (Mogyoros et al., 2000).

2. Conclusion

Paresthesia as one of the presentation of neuropathic pain, had been shown to be caused by different mechanisms. Recent literature were able to elaborate more about the anatomical and physiological basis of paresthesia by using hydroxy-sanshool (sanshool), which is a natural plant alkylamide that induces numbing and robust tingling paresthesia in humans. Sanshool excites specific subtypes of cutaneous mechanoreceptors, it potently activates all ultrasensitive D-hair fibers and, to a lesser extent, unique populations of pressure-sensitive Aß fibers and low conduction velocity C fibers. Paresthesia was seen to be more apparent in rapidly adapting myelinated fibers than the slow one and that has been implicated in both injury- and disease-evoked paresthesia, as well as in post ischemic paresthesia. The cellular and molecular basis of paresthesia is most likely due to two pore potassium channel (KCNK), and not to transient receptor channels (TRPA1). Also, paresthesia generation in the two processes of ischemia and focal nerve compression (FNC) were different. In ischemia, the metabolic byproducts, such as H+, accumulate and potentially interfere with parameters that determine axonal excitability. But during FNC where focal ischaemia appeared to be the underlying mechanism, metabolites exerted less significant effects, as supported by the rapid rate of CSAP recovery observed with release of FNC. More future study is needed in the field of molecular basis of paresthesia, as it seen to be the basis in normal axons in healthy human being.

3. Acknowledgement

I would like to thank my wife and children for their effort, patience and understanding on giving me the time and space to prepare writing this chapter. To Ms. Janice D. Liwanag, for the editing support.

4. References

Al Luwimi, M.; Al Awami, M. (2009). Surgical management of thoracic outlet compression syndrome. Pan Arab Journal of Neurosurgery, Vol. 13, No. 2, (2009), pp. 100-105

Brannagan, T.H.; Lewis, R.P.; Timothy P.A. (2010): Chapter 135, Merritt's Neurology, 12th Edition, Lippincott Williams & Wilkins, pp. 839-843

Han, S.E.; Lin, G.S.Y.; Boland, R.A., et al. (2010): Changes in human sensory axonal excitability induced by focal nerve compression; J Physiol, Vol. 588 No.10 (2010), pp. 1737-1745

Hogan, H.Q. (2007): Role of Decreased Sensory Neuron Membrane Calcium Currents in the Genesis of Neuropathic Pain. Croat Med J, Vol. 48 (2007), pp.j9-21.

Kawasaki, Y.; Zhang, L.; Cheng, J.K., et al. (2008): Cytokine Mechanisms of Central Sensitization: Distinct and Overlapping Role of Interleukin-1_, Interleukin-6, and Tumor Necrosis Factor in Regulating Synaptic and Neuronal Activity in the Superficial Spinal Cord. J. Neurosci.(May 14, 2008), Vol. 28 No. 20, pp. 5189 -5194

Lennertz, R.C.; Tsunozaki, M.; Bautista, M.D. et.al (2010): Physiological Basis of Tingling Paresthesia Evoked by Hydroxy-Sanshool. The Journal of Neuroscience (March 24, 2010), Vol. 30 No. 12, pp. 4353- 4361

Leone, C.; Biasiotta, A; La Cesa, S. et al. (2011): Pathophysiological mechanisms of neuropathic pain. Future Neurology (2011) Vol. 6 No. 4, pp. 497-509

Lewis, R.P. (2005) Chapter 8: Diagnosis of Pain and Paresthesias. Merritt's Neurology 10th Ed; Lewis P. Rowland. 12th Ed. Lippincott, Williams & Wilkins, 2005. pp. 35-38

Mogyoros, I.; Bostock, H.; Burke, D. (2000): Mechanisms of paresthesias arising from healthy axons. Muscle & Nerve (2000) Vol. 23, pp. 310-20

Neil, M.J.E (2011): Acute pain management part 1. Anatomy & Physiology, Anesthesia tutorial of the week. Anatomy & Physiology, 2011; pp. 1-7

Nickel, A.A.(1990). Retrospective Study of Paresthesia of the Dental Alveolar Nerves. Anesth Prog (1990); 37, 42-45.

Roosterman, D.; George, T.; Schneider, S.W,et al. (2006). Neuronal Control of Skin Function: The Skin as a Neuroimmunoendocrine Organ. Physiol Rev (2006) Vol. 86, pp.1309-1379

Ropper A.H.; Samuels, M.A. (2009) Chapter 8. Adams & Victor's Principles of Neurology, 9th Edition, ISBN 978-0-07-149992-7. The McGraw-Hill Companies, Inc. USA

Sindou, M.P.; Mertens, P.; Luis, G.L. (2001) Surgical Procedures for Neuropathic Pain, Neurosurgery Quarterly (March 2001) Vol. 11 No. 1, pp. 45-65

2

Chest Wall Paraesthesia After Thoracic Surgery

Luis Berlanga González, Orlando Gigirey Castro and Sara de Cabanyes Candela
Thoracic Surgery Service, Hospital San Pedro de Alcántara, Cáceres Spain

1. Introduction

Post-operative pain after thoracic surgery is particularly intense and prolonged when compared with other surgical procedures; different stimuli such as rib spreading, costo-chondral dislocation, muscle division, use of diathermy, pleural trauma, pleural drains and subsequent neuroma formation, may play all a part in the development of post-thoracotomy pain.

The origin of pain after thoracic procedures is complex because there is a nociceptive excess carried by somatic and visceral fibers and a major neuropathic component.

According to the IASP (International Association of Pain), the post-thoracotomy pain syndrome is defined as the recurrence or persistence of pain more than two months after thoracotomy, without any recurrence of the disease. Neuropathic features as sensations of dysesthesia, allodynia or burning can be found in 35% to 83% of cases (Maguire et al., 2006).

Dysaesthesia, which is frequently associated with chronic neuropathic pain, can occur in the form of heightened or diminished skin sensation: hypoesthesia (diminished sensation), hypoalgesia (diminished sensation from a painful stimulus), allodynia (pain from a stimulus that is not normally painful) and hyperalgesia (increasing sensation from a painful stimulus). Therefore, dysaesthesia in the early postoperative period may predict chronic pain.

Intercostal nerve damage may cause neuropathic pain through peripheral and central mechanisms. Neuropathic pain is characterized by an area of abnormal pain sensation co-existing with another area of sensory deficit. Often this is accompanied by a hyperpathic state including allodynia and hyperalgesia. Paresthesia has been defined as numbness or disordered sensation causing chest wall discomfort which the patient can distinguish clearly from the wound pain.

Rogers et al., 2000, describes chronic post-thoracotomy pain as a continuous dysaesthetic burning and aching pain in the general area of the incision that persists at least 2 months after thoracotomy. It occurs in approximately 50% of patients after thoracotomy and is usually mild or moderate. However, in 5% of patients is severe and disabling.

Gotoda et al., 2001, studied 85 patients for persistent post-thoracotomy pain; a year after surgery, 35 patients (41.17 %) suffer persistent pain; 24 patients reported paresthesia-dysesthesia and 14 patients complained of hypoesthesia. Clinical time course and symptoms indicate that nerve impairment rather than simple nociceptive impact may be involved in its etiology.

2. Intercostal nerve impairment assessment

The mechanisms producing chronicity in post-thoracotomy acute pain are complex and usually invoke intercostal nerve damage with a central sensitization phenomenon.

Direct injury of the intercostal nerve during thoracic surgery is not needed for symptoms to appear; the use of ratcheted rib spreaders may induce intercostal neuropathy some distance from the surgical site.

Benedetti et al., 1997, assessed intercostal nerve impairment after posterolateral thoracotomy measuring the superficial abdominal reflexes using electrophysiological techniques. They found a close correlation between pain intensity after posterolateral thoracotomy, absence of abdominal reflexes and less effective opioid response; the higher pain intensity with the absence of reflexes may be due to a larger neuropathic component.

Quantitative and selective assessment of intercostal nerve-fiber damage can be tested with a neurometer; current perception threshold values with 2000, 250 and 5 Hz stimuli indicate functions of Aβ, Aδ and C fibers respectively. Aβ fibers are large fibers responsible for touch and pressure sensation. Aδ fibers are small myelinated fibers responsible for sharp pain sensation. C fibers are umyelinated fibers responsible for sensing temperature and dull pain.

Intercostal nerve function was recently assessed (Miyazaki et al., 2011) after three different thoracic surgical procedures: video-assisted thoracic surgery (VATS), video-assisted minithoracotomy with metal retractor and conventional thoracotomy.

VATS group showed no changes in any current threshold values and no residual pain more than 12 weeks after surgery. The video-assisted minithoracotomy with metal retractors group and the conventional thoracotomy group showed significantly higher current perception threshold values at 2000 Hz, 1 week after surgery with pain in approximately 70 % of patients 12 weeks after surgery.

The results of this study showed that the function of myelinated fibers (Aβ and Aδ) was significantly impaired following surgery with metal rib retractors.

Rogers et al., 2002, registred nerve motor evoked potentials intraoperatively in order to identify intercostal nerve injury during thoracotomy; after the rib retractor was removed there was a total conduction block in the nerve immediately above the incision in every patient; if compression and ischaemia is applied to a nerve, neuropraxia will develop at a rate dependent upon severity of the insult.

Neuropraxia will resolve if the compression is removed in a short period of time and the nerve is allowed to recover. However, if the compression persists, then the neuropraxia becomes permanent as the nerve dies and loses its function.

Another intra-operative intercostal nerve conduction study, revealed that nerve injury occurs either as a discrete block at the site of the retractor only, but conducts either side of this point or fails along the whole length of the nerve; These patterns of nerve injury are caused for two different mechanisms of injury: direct pressure on the nerve by the retractor causing a discrete point of trauma that is likely to develop relatively quick, and whilst traction on the nerve causing a much slower onset injury affecting the whole nerve, probably due to ischaemia of the persistently stretched tissues (Maguire et al., 2006).

3. Thoracic surgical procedures

Conventional thoracotomy requires a skin incision greater than 8 cm, either if a posterolateral or an axillary approach was chosen. For the posterolateral incision, the latissimus, trapezius, and rhomboid muscles were divided; for the axillary incision only the serratus anterior muscle was split.

Muscle-sparing thoracotomy technique preserves the latissimus dorsi and serratus anterior muscles; after both muscles attachments are mobilized, latissimus dorsi muscle is retracted posteriorly and serrratus anterior muscle is retracted forward.

Minithoracotomy is a 7-8 cm chest wall incision for video-assisted procedures using several ports, two small metal retractors and a wound retractor.

Video-assisted thoracic surgery (VATS) procedures were performed by visualization through a television monitor; in most cases four or five ports were used and the main skin incision was just 4-5 cm long to remove the lung from the chest cavity with a wound retractor.

Benedetti et al., 1998, analyzed the degree of intercostal nerve impairment comparing posterolateral thoracotomy and muscle-sparing thoracotomy, correlating the nerve damage with long-lasting post-thoracotomy pain. The neurophysiologic recording performed 1 month after either posterolateral or muscle-sparing thoracotomy showed that patients who underwent a posterolateral thoracotomy had a higher degree of intercostal nerve impairment than the muscle sparing thoracotomy patients as revealed by disappearance of the abdominal reflexes, a larger reduction in amplitude of somatosensory-evoked potentials, and a larger increase of the sensory thresholds to electrical stimulation for both tactile perception and pain.

On the other hand, Khan et al., 2000, compared the early and/or late post-operative pain in posterior auscultation triangle thoracotomy incision (muscle-sparing) with full posterolateral thoracotomy (where latissimus dorsi muscle is always cut across its full width). They concluded that early and late post-thoracotomy pain and paraesthesia affecting the area of skin incision and anterior chest wall above and medial to the incision were similar in both incisions.

Similarly, Landreneau et al., 1996, compared the relative efficacies and rates of occurrence of acute or chronic morbidity after muscle-sparing thoracotomy (axillary or lateral) vs. standard lateral thoracotomy. There were no differences between thoracotomy approaches in any of the other primary acute postoperative variables analized (chest tube duration, length of hospital stay, postoperative narcotic requirements, and postoperative mortality).

The frequencies of chronic pain and shoulder dysfunction assessed 1 year after operation were also similar between thoracotomy groups.

Division of serratus anterior and the latissimus dorsi muscles during posterolateral thoracotomy is thought to be related with major postoperative acute and chronic pain.

In muscle-sparing thoracotomy, usually two rib retractors are used instead just one: a small Finochietto rib retractor is positioned within the interspace to widen the intercostal opening; then, a second Finochietto retractor is positioned in a right-angled overlapping fashion with respect to the first retractor to displace the serratus anterior and the latissimus dorsi muscles posteriorly and the pectoralis major muscle anteriorly. During muscle-sparing incisions is necessary to spread the ribs wider apart than in a posterolateral thoracotomy in order to compensate for diminished field of view; in addiction, the use of two rib retractors to displace muscles cause injury to the nerves that would affect muscle function. The most obvious example of this would be injury to the long thoracic nerve, with resulting winged scapula.

3.1 Intercostal nerve protecting surgical techniques

The nerve damage is not significantly associated with most factors except for the technique of closure of the intercostal space: interrupted pericostal sutures are associated with 78% of the low nerve damage and 40% of the high nerve damage.

There are a few prospective studies regarding intercostal nerve protection during thoracotomy closure. Cerfolio et al., 2003, operated on 140 patients who underwent chest closure with pericostal sutures (placed on top of the fifth and seventh ribs) and compared to another 140 patients who underwent chest closure with intracostal sutures (placed on top of the fifth rib and through the small holes drilled in the bed of the sixth rib). They concluded that intracostal sutures were less painful than pericostal sutures, as evaluated at 2 weeks, 1 month, 2 months and 3 month after thoracotomy.

More recently, Bayram et al., 2011, compared two groups of patients who underwent posterior muscle-sparing minithoracotomy in the fifth interspace; in the patients of the group A, two holes were drilled into the sixth rib and sutures were passed through these holes and were circled from the upper edge of the fifth rib, thereby compressing the intercostal nerve underneath the fifth rib. In the group B, the intercostal muscle underneath the fifth rib was partially dissected along with the intercostal nerve, corresponding to the holes on the sixth rib, preventing fifth intercostal nerve compression. Patients of the group B had less post-operative pain as showed lower visual analog scores (VAS) at rest and during coughing.

The conception of a single intercostal nerve running the length of the space is incorrect. Before reaching the angle of the rib, the trunk of the intercostal nerve gives off a branch to the external intercostal muscle and then divides into three main branches:

An upper branch (anterior cutaneous) which occupies the subcostal groove and is the principal or main nerve.

A lower branch which runs for a varying distance along the upper border of the rib below (collateral nerve).

An intermediate, the lateral cutaneous branch, which remains in the deep plane with the other branches until it reaches the level of its exits from the space, where it pierces the internal and external intercostal muscles obliquely (Davies et al, 1932).

In a recent report (McAllister et al, 2011), cadaveric dissections of the 11th intercostal space were performed to characterize intercostal nerve, artery and vein in relationship to the 11th and 12th ribs, in order to access the upper pole of the kidney and realize percutaneous nephrolitostomy. Access placements lateral to the paraspinous muscles and in the lower half of the 11th intercostal space may decrease damage to the intercostal artery and nerve. So far, there are not similar studies in chest wall anatomy to reduce the damage of the intercostal nerves in VATS.

3.2 Video-Assisted Thoracic Surgery

Video-Assisted Thoracic Surgery (VATS) strongly reduces patient postoperative pain, hospital stay and analgesic requirements when compared to open surgery (Hazelrigg et al., 2000); however, over 50% of patients treated by VATS for spontaneous pneumothorax, complain of post-operative chest wall paresthesia related to the portal sites (Sihoe et al., 2004).

In order to improve the results of VATS, smaller instruments and scopes had been used.

Needlescopic instruments (2 mm) have been applied in treating primary spontaneous pneumothorax resulted in better cosmesis and less postoperative pain (Chen et al., 2003).

However, the incidence and nature of paresthesia remains similar even if the level of surgical trauma is further reduced by performing needlescopic VATS. After a needlescopic VATS sympathectomy (T2-T4) for palmar hyperhidrosis study, Sihoe et al., 2005, founded that 50% of patients complained of some type of paresthesic discomfort in the chest: bloating (41.2%), pins and needles (35.5%) or numbness (23.5%).

Moreover, pre-emptive wound infiltration with local anesthetic (0.5% bupivacaine) reduced post-operative wound pain but not reduced chest wall paresthesia in patients who underwent needlescopic VATS sympathectomy for palmar hyperhidrosis (Sihoe et al., 2007).

It may be hypothesized that perhaps the local anesthesia was effective in blocking the sensitization to pain by sharp wound incision, but was less effective in preventing paresthesia which results from blunt trauma and compression to the intercostal nerves.

Although VATS is a minimal invasive surgery procedure, it not eliminates intercostal nerve injury since the scopes are heavily manipulated during procedure, which may cause the nerve to be crushed against the adjacent rib (figure 1).

Nowdays trend in VATS is to use fewer working ports to reduce even more postoperative pain, chest wall paresthesia and hospital stay.

One study compared one and two ports techniques for VATS thoracic sympathectomies; one-port group showed advantages in terms of hospital stay, rate of post-operative pneumothorax and the need for chest drain insertion (Murphy et al., 2006).

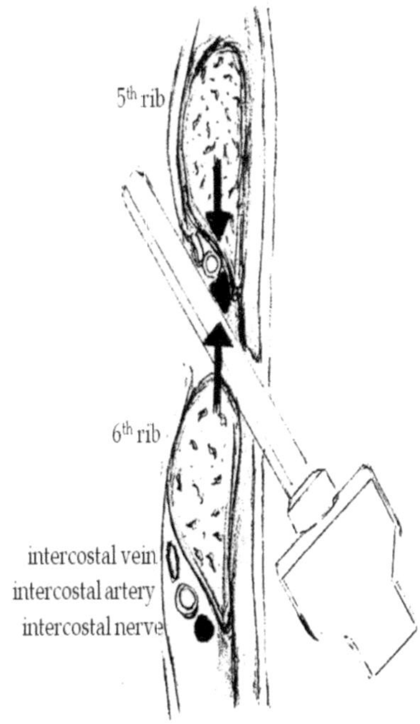

Fig. 1. Intercostal nerve compressed (black arrows) between a rigid port and the 5th rib.

In 1998 was described for the first time the technique of single incision thoracic surgery for pneumothorax in six patients (Yamamoto et al., 1998). The authors were able to introduce a bronchoscope, a grasper and a stapler through a 2 cm long incision in the fifth intercostal space in the midaxillary line.

In other report, single incision VATS technique for spontaneous pneumothorax was used in 16 patients and compared retrospectively to 19 patients who underwent the standard three ports VATS technique; single incision VATS group showed less postoperative pain and lower incidence of residual paresthesias (Jutley et al., 2005).

A prospective no randomized trial, compared 28 patients operated on for spontaneous pneumothorax performing single incision thoracic technique (without protecting sleeves) with23 patients operated on with the standard three port VATS technique; the authors reported no increase of surgical costs, shorter hospital stay and decreased rate of chest wall paraesthesias (35%), in the single incision group (Salati et al., 2008).

The authors (Berlanga & Gigirey, 2011), reported an original technique of uniportal VATS for spontaneous pneumothorax using a single flexible laparoscopic in thirteen patients (Figure 2); three patients (23%) presented mild chest wall paresthesia (numbness); two of them were transient paresthesias and the other one was successfully treated whit a eight-week course of Gabapentin (900 mg/day in 3 doses).

The use of this single flexible port (SILS port™) in VATS procedures protects the intercostal nerves from compression due torquing of the camera or instruments and therefore reduces postoperative pain and rate of residual chest wall paresthesias.

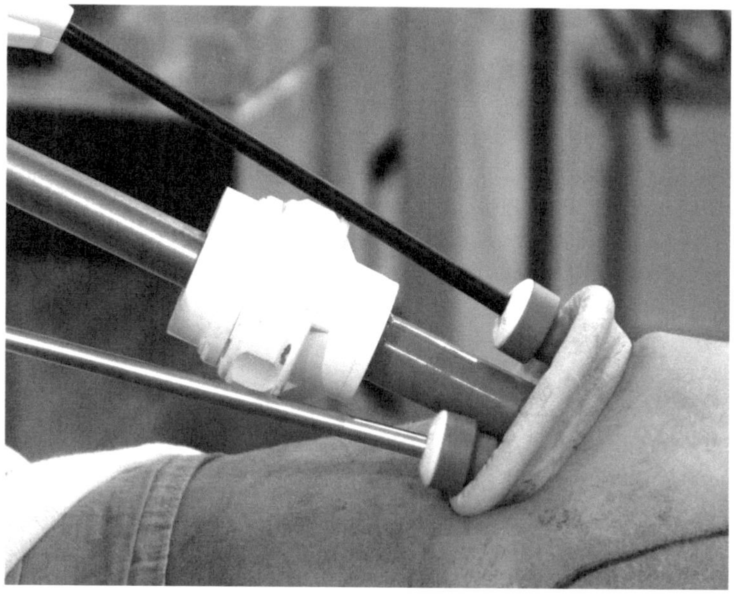

Fig. 2. Thoracoscope, stapler and endograsper introduced through the SILS™ port, lined up along the intercostal space.

Trauma to the intercostal nerves should be minimized by using 5 mm ports for thoracoscope and instruments whenever possible. The long-standing presence of the 10 mm thoracoscope torquing in a small intercostal space could well be responsible for the chronic pain syndrome.

Large port sleeves should be avoided with the only exception to the 12 mm port for the linear stapler; however the stapler does not remain in the intercostal space for any prolonged time.

4. Pre-operative prediction of postoperative chronic pain

Pre-operative pain is one of the best predictors of severe pain in the early post-operative period; a possible explanation for that is that chronic noxious afferent input has produced neuroplastic changes in the spinal cord (sensitization by upregulation of receptor subsystems) that become manifest as relatively hyperpathic state in the post-operative period. One clinical trial has demonstrated that the severe post-operative pain early after awakening from general anesthesia can be predicted at the pre-operative visit with a scoring rule, using the pain domain of the quality of life questionnaire Short form 36 (SF-36) and the Amsterdam Pre-operative Anxiety and information scale (APAIS), (Kalkman et al., 2003).

The transition of acute to chronic post-surgical pain is a complex and poorly understood process, involving biological, psychological and social-environmental factors. Several psychosocial predictors of chronic post-surgical pain have been identified, including increased pre-operative state anxiety, an introverted personality, social support, fear of surgery and "psychic vulnerability", a construct similar to neuroticism (Katz et al., 2009).

5. Pre-emptive analgesia

Maybe the major justification for using pre-emptive anesthesia in thoracic surgery, is the clinical evidence that the decrease in acute post-thoracotomy pain may result in decreased risk of chronic post-thoracotomy pain syndrome.

The factors that affect the transition from acute to chronic pain, were studied in thirty patients who had undergone lateral thoracotomy. Fifty-two percent of these patients reported long-term pain. Early post-operative pain was the only factor that significantly predicted long-term pain. Pain intensity 24 h after surgery, at rest, and after movement, was significantly greater among patients who developed long-term pain compared with pain-free patients (Katz et al., 1996).

Thoracic surgery patients treated with multimodal pre-emptive analgesia with morphine, indomethacin and intercostal nerve blockage with 0.5 % bupivacaine, have shown no differences when comparing to control group in regard to postoperative pain VAS scores, PaCO2 values or postoperative spirometry (Kavanagh et al.,1994).

The pre-emptive effects of administering a 72-h epidural infusion of mepivacaine, beginning before surgery were compared to a postoperative epidural mepivacaine infusion in 70 patients who underwent thoracotomy. Follow-up at 3 and 6 months showed a significant reduction in the incidence of chronic post-thoracotomy pain in the group of patients that received the epidural before surgery (Obata et al.,1999).

Similarly, other authors have found satisfying results with pre-operatively initiated thoracic epidural analgesia in controlling post-thoracotomy pain in the acute and long-term period; they founded decreased incidence and intensity of chronic pain when compared to post-operative epidural or IV analgesia (Sentürk et al., 2002).

Conversely, in another prospective study designed to measure the pre-emptive effect of thoracic epidural analgesia, there was no difference in chronic pain incidence when compared axillary muscle-sparing thoracotomy vs. posterolateral thoracotomy (Ochroch et al., 2005).

Pre-emptive analgesia was intended to prevent the establishment of central sensitization caused by incisional and inflammatory injuries.

The results have not shown a major impact on postoperative pain after thoracic surgery, especially in preventing the development of chronic pain.

A possible explanation for the failure of pre-emptive epidural analgesia in prevent chronic post-thoracotomy pain is that the afferent blockage is not complete, given the variety of incoming stimuli that last for at least several days; in addition, is necessary a complete "humoral blockage" of circulating pro-inflammatory cytokines which lead to central COX-2 induction in the CNS (IL-1β-mediated induction of COX-2), contributing to inflammatory pain hypersensitivity (Gerner et al., 2008).

On the other hand, in neuropathic animal pain models using rib retractors, nearly all myelinated fibers are damaged during the course of allodynia and a extensive Wallerian degeneration was observed 14 days post-surgery; if 0.5 % bupivacaine is given systemically before surgery, mechanical allodynia is prevented (Shin et al., 2008).

This antiallodynic effect of bupivacaine, could be explained by three mechanisms:

First, systemic anti-inflammatory action: after a peripheral nerve injury, the site of damage is typified by the activation of resident immune cells and recruitment and proliferation of nonneuronal elements like neutrophils; a number of soluble mediators can be released (IL-1β) which initiate and maintain sensory abnormalities after injury. Similar to high-dose steroids, which have been proven to contribute to analgesia, local anesthetics including bupivacaine, have been shown to cause anti-inflammatory effects, preventing the release of cytokines.

Secondly, bupivacaine significantly inhibit N-methyl-D-aspartate (NMDA) receptors channel activation, which play an important role in secondary hyperalgesia and chronic pain syndromes.

Finally, subanesthetic doses of local anesthetic drugs, block sodium channel suppressing ectopic electrogenesis and may account for analgesic and antihyperalgesic effects of these drugs.

6. Antiinflamatory drugs

Local tissue damage results in inflammation and propagation of stimuli to the central nervous system. These stimuli are modulated by excitatory (N-methyl-D-aspartate) and inhibitory (opiate) pathways.

Elective surgery provokes an increase in the circulating cytokine levels, especially with regard to interleukin IL-6; the magnitude of the elevation levels is related directly to the degree of tissue injury.

Nagahiro et al. 2001, showed that post-operative pain measurements in VATS patients were significantly less than in posterolateral thoracotomy patients; also the serum interleukin-6 (IL-6) levels in VATS group patients were significantly decreased when compared with IL-6 serum levels in posterolateral thoracotomy group patients. When correlation between pain and cytokines serum levels was studied, a significant correlation was observed with IL-10 in all patients.

Analgesia with anti-inflammatory drugs may contribute to attenuate the postoperative inflammatory response and to prevent postoperative pain in patients undergoing thoracotomy. (NSAIDs) work by inhibiting the cyclooxygenase enzyme responsible for the release of mediators of inflammation.

Patients undergoing thoracotomy showed reduced postoperative pain, reduced analgesic consumption and decreased serum levels of acute phase reactants (IL-6, CPR), when flurbiprofen was added to the systemic analgesic therapy (Esme et al., 2011).

7. Neuropathic pain treatment

Chest wall paresthesia may represent a form of neuropathy following thoracic surgery that requires specific treatment by nonconventional analgesics or opiates drugs.

The prevalence of post-thoracotomy pain syndrome (PTPS) after 12-36 months of follow-up is persistently high; over 40% of patients still use conventional analgesics, but only 2 % use neuropathic medication (Wildgaarg et al., 2010).

7.1 Gabapentin

Gabapentin is an anticonvulsant drug that has antinoceptive and antihyperalgesic properties and is effective in treating chronic neuropathic pain by acting on an specific receptor (alpha 2 delta subunit of presynaptic type N voltage-dependent calcium channels), which are overexpressed in the dorsal horn of the spinal cord and spinal ganglia in cases of neurological injury (Laird et al., 2000).

There is a wide variability in gabapentin regimes depends on: pre-operative, peri-operative or post-operative long-term treatment, type of surgery, type of post-operative rescue analgesic and reported outcomes.

Differences in gabapentin doses as well as frequency of administration will undoubtedly introduce disparity in the pain outcomes.

A single pre-operative dose of gabapentin, 1200 mg or less, effectively reduced pain intensity and opioid consumption for the first 24 h after surgery (Ho et al., 2006).

Turan et al., 2006, used a peri-operative regimen of gabapentin taking 1200 mg pre-operatively, followed by 1200 mg on the morning of the first and second post-operative day.

Others (Fassoulaki et al., 2002) gave their patients 400 mg of gabapentin the night before breast cancer surgery and then 400 mg three times a day for 10 days.

Gabapentin has shown its effectiveness in the treatment of chronic pain after thoracic surgery decreasing, paresthesia around the wound in 75% of cases; 40% of the patients reported at least one minor side effect during treatment (somnolence or dizziness), but only in 6.7% of the patients, gabapentin had to be discontinued because of intolerance of side effects (Sihoe et al., 2006).

Effectiveness of gabapentin was also studied in the treatment of chronic post-throracotomy pain and compared with NSAIDs. Forty patients with posterolateral or lateral thoracotomy were prospectively studied to compare safety and efficacy of gabapentin to naproxen sodium.

Post-operative pain was evaluated by Virtual Analogue Scale (VAS) and the Leeds Assessment of Neuropathic Symptoms and signs (LANSS). At the latest follow up (60th day), the percentage of patients with VAS<5 was 85% in the gabapentin group and 15% in the naproxen group; similarly, the percentage of patients with LANSS score <12 was 85% in the gabapentin group and 0% in the naproxen group (Solak et al., 2007).

Pregabalin is another drug related to Gabapentin, indicated for neuropathic diabetic or postherpetic pain, but is not been well-studied in thoracic surgery patients.

7.2 Capsaicin

Topical capsaicin has been used as treatment for certain neuropathic pain states.

Its mechanism of action appears to be based on selective stimulation of the neurons of amyelinic fibers C, causing the release of substance P, which would disturb pain transmission to central system causing a desensitization phenomenon.

Peripheral neuropathic hypersensitivity is mediated by diverse mechanisms including altered expression of the capsaicin receptor TRPV1 or other key ion channels in affected or intact adjacent peripheral nociceptive nerve fibers, aberrant re-innervation and collateral sprouting, all of which are defunctionalized by topical capsaicin.

However, there are two major limitations to its use. First, modest efficacy of low-concentration capsaicin formulations that are commercially available so far (1% or less), which require repeated daily self-administration. Second, compliance is poor because of intense initial burning effects.

Initial experiences with Capsaicin treatment at high doses (5 - 10 %) require regional anesthesia to tolerate side effects (Robbins et al., 1998).

High dose (8%) concentration of capsaicin patch was recently approved in the EU and USA, a single 60-min application in patients with neuropathic pain produced effective pain relief for up to 12 weeks. Advantages of the high-concentration capsaicin patch include longer duration of effect, patient compliance and low risk for systemic effects or drug–drug interactions (Anad et al., 2011).

8. Myofascial associated pain

Post-operative pain in thoracic surgery is mainly nociceptive; however prolonged central sensitization evidenced as hyperalgesia does occur after surgical trauma and intercostal nerve damage; in addition, nonneuropathic pain can also occur following thoracic surgery.

Hamada et al. 2000, studied several patients with post-operative chronic pain (PTPS) in which myofascial pain was thought to be a causative component of post-thoracotomy pain syndrome. A trigger point in a taut muscular band within the scapular region was founded in 67% of these patients and was effectively treated with injections of 0.5% bupivacaine. The authors recommended that all PTPS patients should be examined in detail to determinate whether there is a trigger point in the scapula region.

9. Surgical treatment for chronic thoracic pain

Patients with chronic post-operative intercostal neuralgia that not response to medical treatment are candidates to surgical neurectomy. A recent study showed a successfully treatment in 5 patients with neurectomy proximal to the intercostal neurinoma of one or more intercostal nerves and implantation of the cut nerve into the latissimus dorsi muscle (Williams et al., 2008).

The site of resection along the course of the intercostal nerves is choosed depending upon the location of the patient´s symptoms and the known anatomy of these nerves; if the patient has a pain in a dermatomal pattern but no motor weakness, it may be possible spare the motor portion of the intercostal nerve by resecting only the perforanting lateral cutaneous branch. If the motor function is nonfunctional or is expendable, then the entire intercostal nerve may be resected proximal to the lesion. If the pain is located only anteriorly, then only the anterior cutaneous branch maybe injured.

For patient who fails to improve after resection of intercostal nerves, there is still the possibility of doing a dorsal gangliectomy.

10. Immunology

Hyperalgesia is commonly found in inflammatory pain conditions where damaged tissue is infiltrated with immune system cells, releasing a variety of soluble mediators that act on peripheral neurons. Allodynia may occur when nerves themselves are damaged (neuropathic pain) which occurs in situations such as diabetic neuropathy, HIV-associated neuropathy, or after surgical trauma.

Many inflammatory mediators (IL-1 and PGE2) act direct on sensory neurons and though cascades of second messengers and kinases, altering the sensitivity of both primary transducing receptors and sodium channels required for action potential transmission.

Pro-inflammatory cytokines can also directly activate and modify gene expression in sensory neurones, and there are several sources of these molecules in close proximity to peripheral nerves. Schwann cells, which have often been thought of having only a passive support role for peripheral nerves, are able to secrete pro-inflammatory cytokines, including via a purinergic P2X7-mediated mechanism (Samad et al., 2001).

Administration of growth factors, such as glial cell line-derived neurotrophic factor (GDNF), could prevent injury-induced transcriptional changes in sensory neurons. Other treatment modalities include the prevention of microglial activation with drugs like minocycline or neuroprotective strategies designed to prevent apoptosis in the dorsal root ganglion or dorsal horn.

Some experimental trials have shown the effects of receptor potential vanilloid 1 (TRPV1) antagonist in regard to improve post-operative analgesia or to reduce the mechanical allodynia.

The analgesic effects of a recently developed transient receptor potential vanilloid 1 (TRPV1) antagonist (AMG0347) were studied in an experimental model of incisional pain (Wu C, et al., 2008). The authors founded that AMG0347 decreased capsaicin-induced heat and mechanical hyperalgesia and blocked central and peripheral TRPV1 receptors. Resiniferatoxin (RTX) is very potent vanilloid receptor against molecularly analogous to capsaicin that causes a slow sustained activation of transient receptor potential vanilloid1 (TRPV-1) receptor.

However, RTX has shown controversial results regarding its use in the treatment of experimental models of chronic pain. Others authors reported that RTX intercostal injections causes a transient hyperalgesic response in injured animals and is ineffective in reducing the mechanical allodynia after thoracotomy (Shin et al., 2010).

11. Genetics

Pain perception is one of the most complicated measurable traits because there is an aggregate of several phenotypes associated with peripheral and central nervous system dynamics, stress responsiveness and inflammatory state.

The manner in which an individual experiences pain and the magnitude of the response to a given pain stimulus may reflect a genetic "set point" in pain sensitivity, irrespective of the degree of tissue damage or inflammation (Diatchenko et al., 2007).

Genetic association studies of pain pathways have complemented the traditional neuroscience approaches of electrophysiology and pharmacology and may point to the novel molecules that mediate neuropathic pain, facilitating its understanding and management.

Recent candidate gene studies have identified and replicated the first associations between several common polymorphisms and pain severity in humans.

Certain allelic variants of the MHC could influence susceptibility to develop and maintain neuropathic pain-like behavior following peripheral nerve injury (Dominguez et al., 2008).

Human genome-wide association studies of pain phenotypes might identify novel analgesic targets, help to prioritize research among current targets, and increase the likelihood of success for analgesics candidates emerging from animal studies.

A range of genetic variations that alter the effectiveness of analgesic drugs, have been identified. In particular, polymorphisms of the cytochrome P450 enzymes (CYP), which play a key role in the metabolism of many drugs, can affect the efficacy of opiates and NSAIDs.

There are some critical regulators of altered pain states, including genes nor normally expressed in the nervous system, but present in cells of the immune system that also are activates in situations of tissue damage. For example, P2RX7, an ATP receptor absent from neurons but present on macrophages and microglia, which is essential for altered inflammatory or neuropathic pain (Foulkes et al., 2008).

In another experimental model of incisional pain, was demonstrated that the heat allodynia and spontaneous firing of impulses in C-fibers innervating the skin adjacent to the incision, depend on Vanilloid 1 transient receptor potential (Trpv1) receptors, and the allodynia and firing of C-fibers were much reduced in Trpv1 gene knockout mice (Banik et al., 2009).

12. Conclusion

The sensation of pain in response to a normal non-painful stimulus (allodynia) or to an exaggerated response to slightly painful stimulus (hyperalgesia), especially when accompanied by numbness, is considered diagnostic for nerve injury.

Although no one thoracic surgical technique has been proved to decrease the incidence of chronic pain, intercostal nerve damage due to rib retraction seems involved in the development of neuralgia.

Video-assisted thoracic surgery reduces postoperative pain, analgesic requirements, hospital stay and the rate of chest paresthesias when compares to open thoracic surgery; residual chest wall paresthesias rate reduces more with the use of flexible ports and uniportal techniques than with the use of needlescopic instruments.

Neuropathic postoperative pain should be identified and treated with anticonvulsant drugs (gabapentin, pregabalin); topical treatment with high dose capsaicin patchs is a value complement.

Future clinical researches in genetics and immunology will help to identify susceptible phenotypes, polymorphisms and allelic variants associated to develop neuropathic pain, as well as, to identify novel analgesic targets to improve postoperative analgesia or to reduce mechanical allodynia.

13. References

Anad P & Bley K. Topical capsaicin for pain manegment: therapeutic potential and mechanism of action of the new high-concentration capsaicin 8% patch. *Br J Anaesth* 2011 Aug 17. (Epub ahead of print).

Bayram AS, Ozcan M, Kaya FN, & Gebitekin C. Rib approximation without intercostal nerve compression reduces post-thoracotomy pain: a prospective randomized study. *Eur J Cardiothorac Surg* 2001;39:570-574.

Benedetti F, Amanzio M, Casadio C, Filosso PL, Molinatti M, Oliaro A, Pischedda F, & Maggi G. Postoperative pain and superficial abdominal reflexes after posterolateral thoracotomy. *Ann Thorac Surg.* 1997;64:207-10.

Benedetti F, Vighetti S, Ricco C, Amanzio M, Bergamasco L, Casadio C, Cianci R, Giobbe R, Oliaro A, Bergamasco B, & Maggi G. Neurophysiologic assessment of nerve impairment in posterolateral and muscle-sparing thoracotomy. *J Thorac Cardiovasc Surg*.1998;115:841- 847.

Berlanga L, & Gigirey O. Uniportal video-assisted thoracic surgery for primary spontaneous pneumothorax using a single-incision laparoscopic surgery port: a feasible and safe procedure. *Surg Endoscopy* 2011;25:2044-2047.

Cerfolio RJ, Price TN, Bryant AS, Bass CS, & Bartolucci AA. Intracostal sutures decreases the pain of thoracotomy. *Ann Thorac Surg* 2003;776:407-412.

Davies F, Gladstone RJ, & Stibbe EP. The anatomy of the intercostal nerves. J Anat 1932;66:323-33.

Diatchenko L, Nackley AG, Tchvileva IE, Shabalina SA, & Maixner W. Genetic Architecture of human pain perception. *Trends Genet* 2007;23:605-607.

Domínguez CA, Lidman O, Hao JX, Diez M, Tuncel J, Olsson T, Wiesenfeld-Hallin Z, Piehl F, & Xu XJ. Genetic analysis of neuropathic pain-like behavior following peripheral nerve injury suggests a role of major histocompatibility complex in development of allodynia. *Pain* 2008;136:313-319.

Esme H, Kesli R, Apillogullari B, Duran FM, & Yoldas B. Effects of Flurbiprofen on CRP, TNF-α, IL-6 and Postoperative Pain of Thoracotomy. *Int J Med* 2011;8:216-221.

Fassoulaki A, Patris k, Sarantopoulos C, & Hogan Q. The analgesic effect of gabapentin and mexiletine after breast surgery for cancer. *Anesth Analg* 2002.;95:985-991.

Foulkes T, & Wood, JN. (2008) Pain Genes. *PLoS Genet* 4: e1000086.

Gerner P. Post-thoracotomy Pain Management Problems. *Anesthesiol Clin* 2008;26:235-367.

Gotoda Y, Kambara N, Sakai T, Kishi Y, Kodama K, & Koyama T. The morbidity, time course and predictive factors for persistent post-thoracotomy pain. *Eur J Pain* 2001:5:89-96.

Hamada H, Moriwaki K, Shiroyama K, Tanaka H, Kawamoto M, & Yuge O. Myofascial pain in patients with postthoracotomy pain syndrome. *Reg Anesth Pain Med* 2000;25:302-305.

Hazelrigg SR, Magee MJ, & Boley TM. (2000). Video-Assisted Spontaneous pneumothorax. In: *Minimal access cardiothoracic surgery*. Yim APC, Hazerlrigg SR, Izatt MB, Landreneau RJ, Mack MJ, Naunheim KS, eds. pp. (73-79). Saunders, Philadelphia, PA.

Ho KY, Gan TJ, & Habib AS. Gabapentin and postoperative pain – a Systematic review of randomized controlled trials. *Pain* 2006;126:91-101.

Jutley RS, Khalil MW, & Rocco G. Uniportal vs. standard three-port VATS technique for spontaneous pneumothorax: comparison of post-operative pain and residual paraesthesia. *Eur J Cardiothorac Surg* 2005;28:43-46.

Kalkman CJ, Visser K, Moen J, & Bonsel DE. Preoperative prediction of severe pain. *Pain* 2003;105:415-423.

Katz J, Jackson M, & Kavanagh BP, et al. Acute pain after thoracic surgery predicts long-term post-thoracotomy pain. *Clin J Pain* 1996;12:50-55.

Katz J, & Seltzer Z. Transition from acute to chronic postsurgical pain: risk factors and protective factors. *Expert Rev Neurother* 2009;9:723-744.

Kavanagh BP, Katz J, Sandler AN, Nierenberg H, Roger S, Boylan JF, & Laws AK. Multimodal analgesia before thoracic surgery does not reduce postoperative pain. *Br J Anaesth* 1994;73:184-189.

Khan IH, McManus KG, McCraith A, & McGuigan JA. Muscle sparing thoracotomy: a biomechanical analysis confirms preservation of muscle strength but no improvement in wound discomfort. *Eur J Cardiothorac Surg* 2000;18:656-661.

Laird MA, & Gidal BE. Use of gabapentin in the treatment of neuropathic pain. *Ann Pharmacother*. 2000;34:802-7.

Landreneau RJ, Pigula F, Luketich JD, Keenan RJ, Bartley S, Fetterman LS, Bowers CM, Weyant RJ, & Ferson P. Acute and chronic morbidity differences between muscle-sparing and standard lateral thoracotomies. *J Thorac Cardiovasc Surg* 1996;112:1346-1351.

Maguire M, Ravenscroft A, Beggs D, & Duffy J. A questionnaire study investigating the prevalence of the neuropathic component of chronic pain after thoracic surgery. *Eur J Cardiothorac Surg*. 2006a;29:800-805.

Maguire MF, Latter JA, Mahajan R, Beggs FD, & Duffy JP. A study exploring the role of intercostals nerve damage in chronic pain after thoracic surgery. *Eur J Cardiothorac Surg* 2006b;29:873-879.

McAllister M, Lim K, Torrey R, Chenoweth J, Barker B, & Baldwin D. Intercostal vessels and nerves are at risk for injury during supracostal percutaneous nephrolitostomy. *J Urol* 2011;185:329- 334.

Miyazaki T, Sakai T, Tsuchiya T, Yamasaki N, Tagawa T, Mine M, Shibata Y, & Nagayasu T. Assessment and follow-up of intercostals nerve damage after video-assisted throracic surgery. *Eur J Thorac Surg* 2011;39:1033-1039.

Murphy MO, Ghosh J, Khwaja N, Murray D, Halka AT, Carter A, Turner NJ, & Walker MG. Upper dorsal endoscopic thoracic sympathectomy: a comparison of one-and two ablation techniques. *Eur J Cardiothorac Surg* 2006;30:223-227.

Nagahiro I, Andou A, Aoe M, Sano Y, Date H, & Shimizu N. Pulmonary function, postoperative pain, and serum cytokine level after lobectomy: a comparison of VATS and conventional procedure. *Ann Thorac Surg* 2001;72:362-365.

Obata H, Saito S, & Fujita N. Epidural block with mepivacaine before surgery reduces long-term post-thoracotomy pain. *Can J Anaesth* 1999; 46:1127–1132.

Ochroch EA, Gottschalk A, Augoustides JG, Aukburg SJ, Kaiser LR, & Shrager JB. Pain and physical function are similar following, muscle-sparing vs. posterolateral thoracotomy. *Chest* 2005;128:2664-2670.

Robbins WR, Staats PS, Levine J, & Fields H. Treatment of intractable pain with topical large-dose Capsaicin: Preliminary report. *Anesth Analg* 1998;86:579-83.

Rogers ML, & Duffy JP. Surgical aspects of chronic post-thoracotomy pain. *Eur J Cardiothorac Surg*. 2000;18:711-6.

Rogers ML, Hendersion L, Mahajan RP, & Duffy JP. Preliminary findings in neurophysiological assessment of intercostal nerve injury during thoracotomy. *Eur J Cardiothorac Surg* 2002;21:298-301.

Salati M, Brunelli A, Xiumè F, Refai M, Sciarra V, Soccetti A, & Sabbatini A. Uniportal video assisted thoracic surgery for primary spontaneous pneumothorax: clinical and economic analysis in comparison to the traditional approach. *Interact Cardiovasc Thorac Surg* 2008;7:63-66.

Samad TA, Moore KA, Sapirstein A, Billet S, Allchrone A, Poole S, Bonventre JV, & Woolf CJ. Interleukin-1beta-mediated induction of Cox-2 in the CNS contributes to inflammatory pain hypersensitivity. *Nature* 2001;410:471-475.

Sentürk M, Ozcan PE, Talu GK, Kiyan E, Cami E, Ozyalcin S, Dilege S, & Pembeci K. The effects of three different analgesia techniques on long-term postthoracotomy pain. *Anesth Analg* 2002;94:11-15.

Shin JW, Pancaro C, Wang CF, & Gerner P. Low-dose systemic bupivacaine prevents the development of allodynia after thoracotomy in rats. *Anesth Analg* 2008;107:1587-1591.

Shin JW, Pancaro C, Wang CF, & Gerner P. The effects of Resiniferatoxin in an experimental rat thoracotomy model. *Anesth Analg* 2010;110:228-232.

Sihoe AD, Au SS, Cheung ML, Chow IK, Chu KM, Law CY, Wan M, & Yim AP. Incidence of chest wall paraesthesia after video assisted surgery for primary spontaneous pneumothorax. *Eur J Cardiovasc Surg* 2004;24:1054-1058.

Sihoe AD, Cheung C, Lai HK, Lee TW, Thung KH, & Yim, A. Incidence of chest wall paresthesia after needlescopic video-assisted thoracic surgery for palmar hyperhidrosis. *Eur J Cardiothorac Surg*. 2005;27:313-319.

Sihoe AD, Lee TW, Wan IY, Thung KH, & Yim AP. The use of gabapentin for post-operative and post-traumatic pain in thoracic surgery patients. *Eur J Cardiothorac Surg* 2006;29:795- 799.

Sihoe AD, Manlulu AV, Lee TW, Wan IY, Thung KH, & Yim AP. Pre-emptive local anesthesia for needlescopic video-assisted thoracic surgery: a randomized controlled trial. *Eur J Cardiothorac Surg* 2007;31:103-108.

Solak O. Merin M & Esme H. Effectiveness of gabapentin in the treatment of chronic post-throracotomy pain. *Eur J Cardiothoracic Surg* 2007;32:9-12.

Wildgaard K, Ravn J, Nikolajsen L, & Jakobsen E. Consequences of persistent pain after lung cancer surgery: a nationwide questionnaire study. *Acta Anaesthesiol Scand* 2010;55:60-68.

Wu C, Gavva NR, & Brennan TJ. Effect of AMG0347, a transient potential type V1 receptor antagonist and morphine on pain behavior after plantar incision. *Anesthesiology* 2008;108:1100-1108.

Yamamoto H, Okada M, Takada M, Mastuoka H, Sakata K, & Kawamura M. Thoracic Surgery Though a Single Skin Incision. *Arch Surg*. 1998;133:145-147.

3

Paraesthesia in Regional Anaesthesia

Bouman Esther, Gramke Hans-Fritz and Marcus A. Marco
Department of Anaesthesiology and Pain Treatment, Maastricht University Medical Centre+, Maastricht, The Netherlands

1. Introduction

Paraesthesia is commonly defined as an abnormal altered sensation ranging from numbness, to burning, tingling or continual pain (Garisto et al. 2010). In regional anaesthesia there should also be "neural" quality as introduction of a needle can induce other causes of pain e.g. skin, tissue or bone contact. So the definition is slightly modified to a burning, shooting or electric sensation or pain usually radiating periferically e.g. to arms, legs or buttocks (Aldrete 2003; Pong et al. 2009).

The aetiology of paraesthesia related to regional anaesthesia is not fully understood. Direct trauma to nerves, local haemorrhage, hydrostatic pressure and neurotoxicity from the local anaesthetic or other injected substances like preservatives and anti-microbial additives may all play a part in the spectrum (Aldrete 2003; Garisto et al. 2010).

During the performance of regional anaesthesia paraesthesia is a frequently reported phenomenon. In the context of paraesthesia two modalities of regional anaesthesia have to be discussed, i.e. the peripheral nerve or conduction block and neuraxial procedures. Both have their own specific clinical indications, applications and complications. Pathophysiology of peripheral nerve injury and spinal cord injury is very similar. However due to the difference in anatomical considerations and applied techniques it will be discussed separately.

2. Peripheral nerve blocks

Peripheral nerve blocks are used to anaesthetize a part of the body, to avoid or complement general anaesthesia and to benefit from good pain relief postoperatively. They can be used for a wide range of unilateral procedures localized a limited body area varying from local eye blocks to regional anaesthesia of upper or lower extremities and even a block of the abdominal wall is possible. These nerve blocks can be performed at any level in the course of a peripheral nerve e.g. the radial nerve can be anaesthetized at the level of the brachial plexus, the elbow or at the wrist, separately or in adjunct to general anaesthesia. Currently there is an increased interest in all kind of new techniques e.g. transverse abdominus plain (TAP), ilioinguinal, iliohypogastric, lumbar plexus, psoas and paravertebral blocks and the continuous use of peripheral nerve catheters in the ambulatory setting is advocated (Lee et al. 2011). Nerve blocks for chronic pain treatment are beyond the scope of this chapter.

2.1 Techniques and approaches localizing peripheral nerves

There are several techniques to localize peripheral nerves: blind techniques, fascial pops, eliciting paraesthesia, trans- and peri-vascular approaches, electrical nerve stimulation, ultrasound/ ultrasonography with or without electrical nerve stimulation, computer tomography (CT) and magnetic resonance imaging (MRI). The first mentioned techniques are frequently used, however in daily clinical practice CT and MRI are nor practically nor workable in the care of the patient (Wedel 2008).

In earlier times elicting paraesthesia was the only way to localize a nerve to perform a peripheral conduction block. Currently more sophisticated techniques are available to clinical practice. Electrical nerve stimulation to elict a motor response of a peripheral nerve is commonly used. However, both techniques are depending on anatomical landmarks and so essentially blind with regard to the nerve itself. The required proximity of the needle to the intended nerve is accompanied by the risk of nerve contact, puncture and damage of related structures. With the use of ultrasound techniques are not blind anymore. Nerves, muscles, blood vessels, pleura and even the spread of local anaesthetic peri-neurally can be visualised (Jeng & Rosenblatt 2011; Marhofer et al. 2010). This does not imply that these techniques are without complications. Although none of the patients suffered from postoperative neurological complications an incidence of unintentional intraneural injection of 17% was reported for ultrasound guided interscalene and supraclavicular nerve blocks (Liu et al. 2011).

There are no safety data available to support one of the mentioned techniques (Chin & Handoll 2011) No technique is proven superior regarding safety and efficacy results are inconsistent (Horlocker 2010). However ultrasounds block peripheral nerve localization showed improved efficacy compared to electrical nerve stimulation techniques in several systematic reviews (Abrahams et al. 2009; Neal, J. M. et al. 2008).

2.2 Paraesthesia and peripheral nerve injury

Fortunately serious neurological complications associated with regional anaesthesia are rare. But this makes it difficult to obtain reliable data about the actual incidence of peripheral nerve block related neurological symptoms. Recent prospective studies reported an incidence of postoperative neurological symptoms between 8-11% direct postoperatively to 0.6% at 6 months (Fredrickson & Kilfoyle 2009; Liu et al. 2009). The majority of the patients reported transient neurological symptoms varying from tingling to paraesthesia resolving between a few days and several months. In France 2.4 serious injuries per 10.000 peripheral nerve blocks were reported (Auroy et al. 2002) It was noted that in case of serious injury or severe neurological complications, they were often related to paraesthesia during needle insertion or pain during injection of the local anesthetics (Auroy et al. 1997). Though permanent neurological injury after a peripheral nerve block is rare neuropathy was reported < 3:100 (Brull et al. 2007). Recently a prospective Australian audit of more than 7000 peripheral nerve and plexus blocks showed and incidence of 0.4 block related nerve injuries per 1000 blocks (Barrington et al. 2009).

2.3 Risk factors for peripheral nerve injury

Risk factors known to be involved in peripheral nerve injury can be divided into patient related, block related and surgery related risk factors.

2.3.1 Patient related risk factors

In general patients who already suffer from medical conditions that affect nerve conduction like multiple sclerosis, diabetic neuropathy, spinal stenosis and lumbar root disease, neurotoxic chemotherapy and patients with peripheral vascular disease are more susceptible to peripheral nerve block related complications. This could be due to increased sensitivity of already damaged nerves or altered blood supply (Horlocker 2010; Jeng et al. 2010). Furthermore some of the patients e.g. obese, pregnant and patients that use potent anti-coagulants are more prone to procedure related technical problems, haematoma and multiple attempts (Brull et al. 2007; Watts & Sharma 2007), which are associated with peripheral nerve injury.

2.3.2 Block related risk factors

Data from the ASA closed claims projects (Lee et al. 2011) show that upper extremity blocks are more associated with claims regarding nerve injuries. The most performed types of peripheral blocks were interscalene and axillary nerve blocks and intravenous regional anaesthesia. The interscalene and axillary blocks were responsible for the majority of the claims (42% and 26 % respectively) (Lee et al. 2011). The brachial plexus was most frequently involved (32%) followed by the median nerve (21%), ulnar nerve (16%), spinal cord (8%) and the phrenic nerve (8%) (Lee et al. 2011). One third of these injuries was permanent and /or disabling (Lee et al. 2011). Spinal cord injuries were all associated with permanent damage and were more frequently related with interscalene blocks under general anesthesia. In 68 % of the claims for nerve injury it was designated as block related. (Lee et al. 2011)

2.3.3 Surgery related risk factors

Surgery related risk factors are ill-defined. However there is an association with trauma. Symptoms can be fracture related e.g. radial nerve injury in proximal humerus fractures or cranial nerve injury after Le Fort I osteotomy (Kim et al. 2011). Furthermore nerve injury is associated with the use of surgical instruments, diathermy, stretch, nerve compression, ischemia, the use of a tourniquet, patient positioning e.g. lithotomy position and peripheral nerve protection. However in what extent which factor contributes to nerve damage is uncertain (Liguori 2004; Watts & Sharma 2007)

2.4 Pathophysiology of peripheral nerve injury

Several mechanisms of nerve injury following surgery under peripheral nerve block have been proposed and described but their relative significance is unknown (Hogan 2008; Liguori 2004).

2.4.1 Neurotoxicity

In cell cultures local anaesthetics in clinically used concentrations cause cytotoxic effects like inhibition of cell growth, necrosis and apoptosis (Hogan 2008). Furthermore local anaesthetics may cause neural membrane lysis due to detergent properties (Kitagawa et al. 2004). The size of these effects is strongly influenced by a prolonged duration of exposure and higher concentration of the local anaesthetics, with in vitro the lowest neurotoxicty for procaine, mepivacaine and lidocaïne compared with ropivacaine and bupivacaine (Hogan 2008; Perez-Castro et al. 2009), however most clinical relevant toxicity is attributed to high concentrations of lidocaïne (Zink & Graf 2003).

In a sciatic nerve rat model direct application of 3% 2-chloroprocaine or 1% tetracaine, but not 2% lidocaïne or 0.75 % bupivacaine resulted in subperineural and endoneural oedema, with mast cell degranulation, proliferation of endoneural fibroblasts, Schwann cell necrosis and axonal dystrophy (Myers et al. 1986). Animal data suggest moreover that amino-ester agents like procaine and tetracaine are more neurotoxic than amino-amide agents like lidocaïne and bupivacaine (Zink & Graf 2003).

Other adjuvants injected together with the local anaesthetic e.g. anti-microbial preservatives added to multi-use vials, anti-oxidants or addition of epinephrine or bicarbonate, may also cause nerve damage (Hogan 2008; Zink & Graf 2003).

2.4.2 Mechanical nerve damage

Nerve injury from nerve contact or penetration is more likely to result due to sharp-bevelled needles than to blunt bevelled needles. However needle-tip penetration is not always the cause of nerve injury. Penetration of fascicles with or without infusion of saline did not result in changes in microscopy or alterations of diffusion barriers, despite high infusion pressures (Hogan 2008). But nerves are not homogenous structures so it is possible to penetrate a nerve without reaching and damaging a neuronal structure.

High injection pressures moreover are associated with persistent neurological deficits after intra neural injections indicating that the surrounding perineurium is very important to protect the fascicles from the cytotoxic effects of the local anaesthetics (Hogan 2008; Jeng & Rosenblatt 2011).

It remains unclear whether a block technique to elict paraesthesia increases the risk of peripheral nerve injury (Horlocker 2001). Nevertheless peripheral nerve damage remains associated with injection of local anaesthetic and paraesthesia or pain on injection of a local anaesthetic (Auroy et al. 2002; Hogan 2008).

Other mechanisms of mechanical nerve damage include surgical trauma, peri- and post-operative positioning and damage from tourniquets. If the latter is a result of ischemia or mechanical deformation is unclear. However by compression of the nerve under the edge of a pneumatic cuff substantial distortion of myelin lamellae and axonal shrinkage is reported as early as 2-4 hours after tourniquet inflation (Hogan 2008; Liguori 2004).

2.4.3 Ischemia

The earliest response to ischemia of a peripheral neuron is depolarisation and spontaneous activity, perceived by the patient as paraesthesia. Nerve function is restored completely after ischemia of less than 2 hours and ischemic periods to up to 6 hours failed to produce permanent structural nerve changes. However histological examination showed oedema and fiber degeneration (Hogan 2008). Ischemic injury may result from pressure and volume of the local anesthetic or added vasoconstrictors. Moreover local anaesthetics like lidocaïne and bupivacaine decrease neuronal blood flow. However contribution of vasoconstriction to peripheral nerve injury has not been proved (Hogan 2008).

Haematoma and vascular injury are difficult to classify as they may cause local ischemia but may provoke local high pressures as well (Liguori 2004).

2.5 Diagnosis and management of peripheral nerve injury

The best treatment of neurological deficit is prevention and starts with a good pre-operative preparation and complete documentation of the block. This includes information about the pre-existent condition of the patient, concomitant diseases, used techniques, local anaesthetics and adjuvants used, complications or difficulties during the procedure, the efficacy and the duration of the block and the surgical procedure. Direct postoperative follow-up should be performed in all patients. If symptoms occur careful physical examinations should be performed and an expert e.g. neurologist should be consulted. Electrophysiological testing should be performed to define a neurogenic basis of nerve damage, to localize the site of injury and to define the severity of the injury.

If compression is suspected ultrasonography or an MRI of the plexus has to be done. (Borgeat 2005; Mayfield 2005; Neal, J. M. et al. 2008)

3. Neuraxial block

Neuraxial blocks are applied to induce anaesthesia or analgesia in a limited part of the body. Especially patients scheduled for major thoracic or abdominal procedures or procedures in the lower extremities or pelvis can benefit from these techniques.

There are 3 techniques to provide neuraxial blockade: Spinal, epidural and a combination of both for longer lasting analgesia i.e. combined spinal-epidural anaesthesia (CSE) as a needle through needle procedure or with the insertion of a catheter at a different level (Warren 2008).

Spinal or dural anaesthesia implies perforation of the dura and arachnoid matter, and after aspiration of cerebrospinal fluid, injection of local anaesthetic. Whereas in epidural anaesthesia the dura remains intact. Spinal anaesthesia is restricted to the lumbar region due to the presence of the conus medullaris at the level of L1-L2 in the adult, but a wide variation exists between as high as T12 to as low as L4. Especially in patients with difficult surface landmarks these anatomical variations can lead to more cephalad needle placement than intended (Neal, J.M 2008). However recently experimental higher spinal techniques are described in literature (van Zundert et al. 2007).

The epidural space can be accessed at any level up to C7 to induce a segmental anaesthetic block depending on the site of injection of local anaesthetics (Warren 2008). The technique relies on anatomical landmarks for penetration of the ligamentum flavum to localize the epidural space. The ligamentum flavum however fuses not always in the midline, especially in the upper thoracic en cervical levels. Moreover the depth of the epidural space itself decreases from 5-8 mm in the lumbar region to 1-2 mm in the upper thoracic and cervical regions (Neal, J.M 2008).

3.1 Paraesthesia and the neuraxial block

In contrast to the peripheral conduction block elicting paraesthesia for neuraxial block is never aimed for. As there are no nerve roots in the posterior epidural space the occurrence of paraesthesia implies perforation of the dural sac with direct contact or puncture of the spinal cord, intrathecal contact with nerve roots, or, more frequently, extradurally contact with an exciting nerve root. Paraesthesia usually does not lead to neurological sequelae but is an unpleasant sensation for the patient and the significance still remains unclear (Aldrete 2003; Neal, J.M 2008).

3.2 Paraesthesia and spinal, epidural and combined spinal epidural anaesthesia

Reported incidences of paraesthesia vary between 0.2 and 56% depending on approach (Leeda et al. 2005), patient characteristics (Hebl et al. 2010; Spiegel et al. 2009), technique (Hebl et al. 2006; McAndrew & Harms 2003; van den Berg et al. 2011), different catheters (Bouman et al. 2007; Jaime et al. 2000)and depth of insertion (Cartagena & Gaiser 2005). Even an incidence as high as 81% -89% was reported (Hetherington et al. 1994; van den Berg et al. 2005).

The symptoms of paraesthesia during conduct of neuraxial anaesthesia are frequently mild and transient. However sometimes they are so intense that the procedure must be aborted. Fortunately the incidence of permanent neurological damage of 1:20.000-30.000 for spinal anaesthesia and 1:25.000 for obstetric epidurals and 1:3600 in other epidurals remains low (Moen et al. 2004), but in France two thirds of the patients with neurological deficits reported paraesthesia during needle placement or pain on injectionof local anaesthetics (Auroy et al. 1997).

Moreover it seems that paraesthesia is like pre-existing neurological disease, degenerative spinal disease, obesity, female sex and anti-coagulation a risk factor for or an indicator of a complicated procedure and therefore for permanent neurological injury (Aldrete 2003; Brull et al. 2007; Fowler 2007).

3.3 Transient neurological symptoms

Transient neurological symptoms (TNS) were first reported in 1993. After an uneventful spinal anaesthesia and after full recovery, within a few hours symptoms of light to severe pain in the gluteal region (buttocks) radiating to both lower extremities start with a duration of 6 hours up to 5 days. Furthermore no abnormalities on neurological examination, MRI or electrophysiological testing should be demonstrated (Pollock 2003; Zaric & Pace 2009).

The highest incidences of TNS are found in patients with intrathecal lidocaïne undergoing surgery in lithotomy position (30-36%), arthroscopic knee surgery (18-22%), while in patients undergoing other surgery in supine position the incidences are 4-8% (Pollock 2003).

Although interpreted as possible neurotoxicity of lidocaine TNS is associated with all other local anaesthetics however in a lower incidence (Zaric & Pace 2009). Decreasing lidocaïne concentration from 5 to 0.5 % does not decrease the incidence of TNS. Glucose, hyperbaricity and hyperosmolarity are not contributing factors (Pollock 2003).

Other possible causes are direct needle trauma, neural ischemia secondary to sciatic stretching, patient positioning, pooling of local anaesthetics, muscle spasm, early mobilization and irritation of the dorsal root ganglion (Pollock 2003).

Treatment can be very difficult. In general non-steroidal anti-inflammatory drugs are prescribed; occasionally opioids are necessary to treat the symptoms. Prevention is essential as treatment is not always successful. If neurological examination is abnormal other possible complications have to be ruled out e.g. epidural haematoma or nerve root damage (Pollock 2003).

3.4 Serious neurological complications

Although rare, if neurological deficits occur serious complications have to be ruled out. Most cases of spinal haematoma are characterized by an acute or subacute course with acute onset of pain at the level of the haemorrhage with more or less severe paralysis with or without bladder/intestinal disturbances (Kreppel et al. 2003).

Direct neurological or neurosurgical consultation, MRI and neurophysiolocal testing is required because possible treatment options. Decompressive laminectomy for epidural haematoma, antibiotics and possible surgical drainage for epidural abscess and meningitis, hypertensive therapy for anterior spinal artery syndrome are necessary to reduce morbidity.

A decompressive laminectomy should be done within 6-8 hours after start of the symptoms to avoid permanent spinal cord injury (Kreppel et al. 2003; Neal, J. M. et al. 2008). For spinal nerve injury, adhesive arachnoiditis and cauda equine syndrome no effective treatment is available (Naguib et al. 1998; Pollock 2003).

Epidural abscess and meningitis are not further discussed as there no obvious relation with paraesthesia.

3.5 Pathophysiology of spinal cord, spinal root and spinal nerve injury

Like peripheral nerve injury spinal cord and spinal root injury after the conduct of a neuraxial block has several proposed mechanisms. Sometimes the mechanism is obvious like in case of epidural haematoma, but often the cause of spinal cord injury remains unclear of multifactorial.

3.5.1 Mechanical injury of the spinal cord and spinal nerve damage

Mechanical injury of the spinal cord and spinal nerves during of after conduct of a neuraxial block can be caused by several mechanisms.

The vertebral column protects spinal cord and spinal nerves to mechanical injury. To perform a neuraxial block it is necessary to precisely avoid this defence. The access to the spinal canal is based on landmark techniques, but ultrasound becomes more common practice (Balki 2010; Perlas 2010). However as earlier indicated human anatomy varies and this can lead to failure to contact identifiable landmarks, unintentional cephalad needle placement, and unintentional penetration of the dura.

Penetration of the spinal cord can provoke intense pain, pressure or paraesthesia or no sensation at all. After penetration of the spinal cord, damage can occur from injury of neural structures, haematoma, oedema, central syrinx creation, local anaesthetic or adjuvant toxicity or a combination of these factors (Neal, J.M 2008).

Furthermore reduction of the vertebral canal diameter by degenerative changes, intra- and extradural mass lesions e.g. haematoma, and patient positioning may compromise spinal cord blood flow. This by increasing spinal cord or CSF pressure, decreasing arterial inflow and venous outflow leading to spinal cord ischemia, possibly worsened by injected or infused local anaesthetic (Neal, J.M 2008).

3.5.2 Vascular injury

The spinal cord and cauda equine receive two thirds of their blood supply from the anterior spinal artery (ASA). The lower thoracic and lumbar sacral spinal cord are supplied by the arteria radicularis magna or artery of Adamkiewicz which provides 25-50% of the total spinal cord blood flow (Biglioli et al. 2004; Neal, J.M 2008). Spinal cord blood flow is like the cerebral blood flow auto regulated with mean arterial pressures between 50/60 - 120 mmHg in animal models and hypoperfusion with hypo perfusion is an often suggested cause of spinal cord damage. However in patients undergoing spine surgery prolonged periods of hypotension induced no detectable spinal cord injury, nor is anterior spinal artery syndrome associated with cardiopulmonary bypass or induced hypotension. Nevertheless the diagnosis anterior spinal artery syndrome has been made in cases with unexplained injury associated with neuraxial blocks. Underlying medical conditions like atherosclerosis are more probable explanations than hypotension or vasoactive agents (Neal, J.M 2008).

Direct vascular trauma from midline and paramedian approaches is anatomically unlikely, but possible during lateral or peri-spinal approaches as psoas compartment or celiac plexus blocks, but no human data supports this view (Neal, J.M 2008).

3.5.3 Neurotoxicity

As earlier mentioned all local anaesthetics have the potential of neurotoxicity. However in clinically used doses local anaesthetics, opioids, adjuvants and preservatives are relatively safe (Hodgson et al. 1999). However after disruption of the blood-spinal cord barrier certain anatomic conditions may contribute to increased susceptibility to injury. The cauda equina consists of partly unmyelinated nerve fibres with a relative high surface area which is exposed to potentially neurotoxic agents. Secondly, nerve roots in the blood-spinal cord barrier lack connective tissue which provides mechanical and metabolic protection compared with peripheral nerves. Furthermore clearance of toxic substances by CSF is not as efficient as vascular clearance which causes spinal cord and spinal nerve roots to be exposed to drug maldistribution and local high drug doses. These factors are believed to have contributed to cases with cauda equina syndrome after spinal anaesthesia with micro catheters (Neal, J.M 2008).

4. Conclusions

During the conduct of regional anaesthesia paraesthesia is a frequently reported phenomenon. It is a risk factor for or an identifier of a complicated procedure and in such a way for permanent neurological injury. Other risk factors are patient, procedure or block related. Possible causes of neurological injury are mechanical, vascular or ischemia and neurotoxicity.

Although rare, if neurological deficits occur serious complications have to be ruled out, by neurological or neurosurgical consultation, and neurophysiolocal testing. This because possible treatment options have to be enforced as soon as possible to minimize morbidity. MRI is the preferred mode of imaging to demonstrate spinal canal pathology. The best treatment of neurological deficit is prevention and starts with a good pre-operative preparation and complete documentation of the block.

5. Acknowledgements

The authors would like to thank Mrs. Resy VanderBroeck for her valuable comments and preparation of the manuscript.

6. References

Abrahams, M.S., M.F. Aziz, R.F. Fu & J.L. Horn (2009). "Ultrasound guidance compared with electrical neurostimulation for peripheral nerve block: a systematic review and meta-analysis of randomized controlled trials." *Br J Anaesth* 1023 (3Mar): 408-417

Aldrete, J.A. (2003). "Neurologic deficits and arachnoiditis following neuroaxial anesthesia." *Acta Anaesthesiol Scand* 471 (1Jan): 3-12

Auroy, Y., D. Benhamou, L. Bargues, C. Ecoffey, B. Falissard, F.J. Mercier, H. Bouaziz & K. Samii (2002). "Major complications of regional anesthesia in France: The SOS Regional Anesthesia Hotline Service." *Anesthesiology* 975 (5Nov): 1274-1280

Auroy, Y., P. Narchi, A. Messiah, L. Litt, B. Rouvier & K. Samii (1997). "Serious complications related to regional anesthesia: results of a prospective survey in France." *Anesthesiology* 873 (3: 479-486

Balki, M. (2010). "Locating the epidural space in obstetric patients-ultrasound a useful tool: continuing professional development." *Can J Anaesth* 5712 (12Dec): 1111-1126

Barrington, M.J., S.A. Watts, S.R. Gledhill, R.D. Thomas, S.A. Said, G.L. Snyder, V.S. Tay & K. Jamrozik (2009). "Preliminary results of the Australasian Regional Anaesthesia Collaboration: a prospective audit of more than 7000 peripheral nerve and plexus blocks for neurologic and other complications." *Reg Anesth Pain Med* 346 (6Nov-Dec): 534-541

Biglioli, P., M. Roberto, A. Cannata, A. Parolari, A. Fumero, F. Grillo, M. Maggioni, G. Coggi & R. Spirito (2004). "Upper and lower spinal cord blood supply: the continuity of the anterior spinal artery and the relevance of the lumbar arteries." *J Thorac Cardiovasc Surg* 1274 (4Apr): 1188-1192

Borgeat, A. (2005). "Neurologic deficit after peripheral nerve block: what to do?" *Minerva Anestesiol* 716 (6Jun): 353-355

Bouman, E.A., H.F. Gramke, N. Wetzel, T.H. Vanderbroeck,R. Bruinsma,M. Theunissen,H.E. Kerkkamp & M.A. Marcus (2007). "Evaluation of two different epidural catheters in clinical practice. narrowing down the incidence of paresthesia!" *Acta Anaesthesiol Belg* 582 (2: 101-105

Brull, R., C.J. McCartney, V.W. Chan & H. El-Beheiry (2007). "Neurological complications after regional anesthesia: contemporary estimates of risk." *Anesth Analg* 1044 (4Apr): 965-974

Cartagena, R. & R.R. Gaiser (2005). "Advancing an epidural catheter 10 cm then retracting it 5 cm is no more effective than advancing it 5 cm." *Journal of clinical anesthesia* 177 (72005/11): 528-530

Chin, K.J. & H.H. Handoll (2011). "Single, double or multiple-injection techniques for axillary brachial plexus block for hand, wrist or forearm surgery in adults." *Cochrane Database Syst Rev* 7: CD003842

Fowler, S.J. (2007). "Risk of a severe neurological complication after regional anesthesia should be individualized." *Anesth Analg* 1053 (3Sep): 880-881; author reply 881

Fredrickson, M.J. & D.H. Kilfoyle (2009). "Neurological complication analysis of 1000 ultrasound guided peripheral nerve blocks for elective orthopaedic surgery: a prospective study." *Anaesthesia* 648 (8Aug): 836-844

Garisto, G.A., A.S. Gaffen, H.P. Lawrence, H.C. Tenenbaum & D.A. Haas (2010). Occurrence of Paresthesia After Dental Local Anesthetic Administration in the United States. 141: 836-844.

Hebl, J.R., T.T. Horlocker, S.L. Kopp & D.R. Schroeder (2010). "Neuraxial blockade in patients with preexisting spinal stenosis, lumbar disk disease, or prior spine surgery: efficacy and neurologic complications." *Anesth Analg* 1116 (6Dec): 1511-1519

Hebl, J.R., S.L. Kopp, D.R. Schroeder & T.T. Horlocker (2006). "Neurologic complications after neuraxial anesthesia or analgesia in patients with preexisting peripheral sensorimotor neuropathy or diabetic polyneuropathy." *Anesth Analg* 1035 (5Nov): 1294-1299

Hetherington, R., R.A. Stevens, J.L. White, L. Spitzer & S. Koppel (1994). "Subjective experiences of anesthesiologists undergoing epidural anesthesia." *Reg Anesth.* 194 (4: 284-288.

Hodgson, P.S., J.M. Neal, J.E. Pollock & S.S. Liu (1999). "The neurotoxicity of drugs given intrathecally (spinal)." *Anesth Analg* 884 (4Apr): 797-809

Hogan, Q.H. (2008). "Pathophysiology of peripheral nerve injury during regional anesthesia." *Reg Anesth Pain Med* 335 (5Sep-Oct): 435-441

Horlocker, T.T. (2001). "Neurologic complications of neuraxial and peripheral blockade." *Canadian Journal of Anesthesia* 48S1 (S1: R72-76

Horlocker, T.T. (2010). "Complications of regional anesthesia." *European Journal of Pain Supplements* 44 (4: 227-234

Jaime, F., G.L. Mandell, M.C. Vallejo & S. Ramanathan (2000). "Uniport soft-tip, open-ended catheters versus multiport firm-tipped close-ended catheters for epidural labor analgesia: a quality assurance study." *J Clin Anesth* 122 (2Mar): 89-93

Jeng, C.L. & M.A. Rosenblatt (2011). "Intraneural injections and regional anesthesia: the known and the unknown." *Minerva Anestesiol* 771 (1Jan): 54-58

Jeng, C.L., T.M. Torrillo & M.A. Rosenblatt (2010). "Complications of peripheral nerve blocks." *Br J Anaesth* 105 Suppl 1Dec): i97-107

Kim, J.W., B.R. Chin, H.S. Park, S.H. Lee & T.G. Kwon (2011). "Cranial nerve injury after Le Fort I osteotomy." *Int J Oral Maxillofac Surg* 403 (3Mar): 327-329

Kitagawa, N., M. Oda & T. Totoki (2004). "Possible mechanism of irreversible nerve injury caused by local anesthetics: detergent properties of local anesthetics and membrane disruption." *Anesthesiology* 1004 (4Apr): 962-967

Kreppel, D., G. Antoniadis & W. Seeling (2003). "Spinal hematoma: a literature survey with meta-analysis of 613 patients." *Neurosurg Rev* 261 (1Jan): 1-49

Lee, L.A., K.L. Posner, C.D. Kent & K.B. Domino (2011). "Complications Associated With Peripheral Nerve Blocks: Lessons From the ASA Closed Claims Project." *Int Anesthesiol Clin* 493 (3Summer): 56-67

Leeda, M.,R. Stienstra, M.S. Arbous, A. Dahan, B. Th Veering, A.G. Burm & J.W. Van Kleef (2005). "Lumbar epidural catheter insertion: the midline vs. the paramedian approach." *Eur J Anaesthesiol* 2211 (11Nov): 839-842

Liguori, G.A. (2004). "Complications of regional anesthesia: nerve injury and peripheral neural blockade." *J Neurosurg Anesthesiol* 161 (1Jan): 84-86

Liu, S.S., J.T. YaDeau, P.M. Shaw, S. Wilfred, T. Shetty & M. Gordon (2011). "Incidence of unintentional intraneural injection and postoperative neurological complications with ultrasound-guided interscalene and supraclavicular nerve blocks." *Anaesthesia* 663 (3Mar): 168-174

Liu, S.S., V.M. Zayas, M.A. Gordon, J.C. Beathe, D.B. Maalouf, L. Paroli, G.A. Liguori, J. Ortiz, V. Buschiazzo, J. Ngeow, T. Shetty & J.T. Ya Deau (2009). "A prospective, randomized, controlled trial comparing ultrasound versus nerve stimulator guidance for interscalene block for ambulatory shoulder surgery for postoperative neurological symptoms." *Anesth Analg* 1091 (1Jul): 265-271

Marhofer, P., H. Willschke & S. Kettner (2010). "Current concepts and future trends in ultrasound-guided regional anesthesia." *Curr Opin Anaesthesiol* 235 (5Oct): 632-636

Mayfield, J.B. (2005). "Diagnosis and management of peripheral nerve block complications." *Int Anesthesiol Clin* 433 (3Summer): 119-126

McAndrew, C.R. & P. Harms (2003). "Paraesthesiae during needle-through-needle combined spinal epidural versus single-shot spinal for elective caesarean section." *Anaesthesia and intensive care* 315 (5Oct): 514-517

Moen, V., N. Dahlgren & L. Irestedt (2004). "Severe neurological complications after central neuraxial blockades in Sweden 1990-1999." *Anesthesiology* 1014 (4Oct): 950-959

Myers, R.R., M.W. Kalichman, L.S. Reisner & H.C. Powell (1986). "Neurotoxicity of local anesthetics: altered perineurial permeability, edema, and nerve fiber injury." *Anesthesiology* 641 (1Jan): 29-35

Naguib, M., M.M. Magboul, A.H. Samarkandi & M. Attia (1998). "Adverse effects and drug interactions associated with local and regional anaesthesia." *Drug Saf* 184 (4Apr): 221-250

Neal, J.M. (2008). "Anatomy and pathophysiology of spinal cord injury associated with regional anesthesia and pain medicine." *Reg Anesth Pain Med* 335 (5Sep-Oct): 423-434

Neal, J.M., C.M. Bernards, A. Hadzic, J.R. Hebl, Q.H. Hogan, T.T. Horlocker, L.A. Lee, J.P. Rathmell, E.J. Sorenson, S. Suresh & D.J. Wedel (2008). "ASRA Practice Advisory on Neurologic Complications in Regional Anesthesia and Pain Medicine." *Regional Anesthesia and Pain Medicine* 335 (52008/10//): 404-415

Perez-Castro, R.,S. Patel, Z.V. Garavito-Aguilar, A. Rosenberg, E. Recio-Pinto, J. Zhang, T.J. Blanck & F. Xu (2009). "Cytotoxicity of local anesthetics in human neuronal cells." *Anesth Analg* 1083 (3Mar): 997-1007

Perlas, A. (2010). "Evidence for the use of ultrasound in neuraxial blocks." *Reg Anesth Pain Med* 352 Suppl (2 SupplMar-Apr): S43-46

Pollock, J.E. (2003). "Neurotoxicity of intrathecal local anaesthetics and transient neurological symptoms." *Best Practice & Research Clinical Anaesthesiology* 173 (3: 471-484

Pong, R.P., B.S. Gmelch & C.M. Bernards (2009). "Does a paresthesia during spinal needle insertion indicate intrathecal needle placement?" *Reg Anesth Pain Med* 341 (1Jan-Feb): 29-32

Spiegel, J.E., A. Vasudevan, Y. Li & P.E. Hess (2009). "A randomized prospective study comparing two flexible epidural catheters for labour analgesia." *Br J Anaesth* 1033 (3Sep): 400-405

van den Berg, A.A., S. Ghatge, G. Armendariz, D. Cornelius & S. Wang (2011). "Responses to dural puncture during institution of combined spinal-epidural analgesia: a comparison of 27 gauge pencil-point and 27 gauge cutting-edge needles." *Anaesth Intensive Care* 392 (2Mar): 247-251

van den Berg, A.A., M. Sadek, S. Swanson & S. Ghatge (2005). "Epidural injection of lidocaine reduces the response to dural puncture accompanying spinal needle insertion when performing combined spinal-epidural anesthesia." *Anesth Analg* 1013 (3Sep): 882-885, table of contents

van Zundert, A.A., G. Stultiens, J.J. Jakimowicz, D. Peek, W.G. van der Ham, H.H. Korsten & J.A. Wildsmith (2007). "Laparoscopic cholecystectomy under segmental thoracic spinal anaesthesia: a feasibility study." *Br J Anaesth* 985 (5May): 682-686

Warren, D., Liu SS (2008). Neuraxial anesthesia in *Anesthesiology*. B. D. DE Longnecker, Newman MF , Zapol WM,978-1008,The McGraw-Hill Companies, ISBN 978 0 07 148995 9,New York, USA

Watts, S.A. & D.J. Sharma (2007). "Long-term neurological complications associated with surgery and peripheral nerve blockade: outcomes after 1065 consecutive blocks." *Anaesth Intensive Care* 351 (1Feb): 24-31

Wedel, D.J., Horlocker T.T (2008). Peripheral nerve blocks in *Anesthesiology*. B. D. D. E Longnecker, Newman MF , Zapol WM,1025-1052,The McGraw-Hill Companies, ISBN 978 0 07 148995 9,New York, USA

Zaric, D. & N.L. Pace (2009). "Transient neurologic symptoms (TNS) following spinal anaesthesia with lidocaine versus other local anaesthetics." *Cochrane Database Syst Rev*2 (2: CD003006

Zink, W. & B.M. Graf (2003). "[Toxicology of local anesthetics. Clinical, therapeutic and pathological mechanisms]." *Anaesthesist* 5212 (12Dec): 1102-1123

4

Paresthesia in Spinal Anesthesia

Luiz Eduardo Imbelloni and Marildo A. Gouveia
Faculty of Medicine Nova Esperança FAMENE,
João Pessoa, PB,
Brazil

1. Introduction

Spinal anesthesia is induced by injecting small amounts of local anesthetic into the cerebro-spinal fluid (CSF), which solution must be capable of blocking nerve paths, and non-toxic, that is, it should not hinder the proper functioning of the bulbar centers, or interfere with the metabolic processes of the more important organs. The injection is usually made in the lumbar spine below the level at which the spinal cord ends (L_2). Recently the anatomy of the thoracic spinal canal was investigated with magnetic resonance image (RMI) 19 [1] and 50 [2] patients, and it has been demonstrated the safety of the segmental spinal anesthesia at T10 by using the combined spinal-epidural technique [3] or single puncture [4].

If the anesthetist has an adequate knowledge of the relevant anatomy, physiology and pharmacology, safe and satisfactory anesthesia can easily be obtained to the mutual satisfaction of the patient, surgeon and anesthetist. To become expert in the art of spinal anesthesia is no simple matter for the beginner, for many solutions and techniques are available and many problems present themselves which form subjects for discussion and disagreement. The literature is abundant, very illuminating and worthy of very close inspection for begin. Direct trauma to nervous tissue may occur at the level of the spinal cord, nerve root, or peripheral nerve. During attempts to insert a spinal needle into the subarachnoid space, patients occasionally experience paresthesia with a report ranging from 6.3% to 20% [5-8]. Two thirds of anesthesia related neurological complications are associated with either paresthesia (direct nerve trauma) or pain during injection (intraneural location) [9]. Although the etiology of paresthesia has not been precisely determined, the widely held conventional wisdom is that they result from needle to nerve contact. Some anesthesiologists believe paresthesias occur when the needle contacts a spinal nerve within the epidural space or the subarachnoid space and as such indicates that spinal needle is misdirected. Because of this, several authors advocate withdrawing the spinal needle and redirecting it away from side where the paresthesia occurred [5-9].

2. Definition

Paresthesia during regional anesthesia is an unpleasant sensation for patients and, more importantly, in some cases it is related to neurological injury. Paresthesia is an abnormal condition in which patients feel a sensation of burning, numbness, tingling, itching or prickling. Paresthesia can also be described as a pins-and-needles or skin-crawling sensation. Paresthesia most often occurs in the extremities, such as the hands, feet, fingers, and toes, but it can occur in other parts of the body. Paresthesia during spinal anesthesia increases patient discomfort and the risk of abrupt movement but, more importantly, paresthesia may be associated with neurological damage. The sensation is unpleasant and it usually has two phases: the first one is the sudden excitation of the muscle involved with that nerve if it is a motor one (fast conduction). And second, one form of pain sensation if the fibers are of a sensitive nerve (slow conduction). In the mixed nerves the shock dominates the sensation. The consequences may be none or, if confirmed, resolved by time in the benign cases, eventually with the aid of physiotherapy, or it may leave a sequel after the treatment. The sequel is usually reduced strength or impotence because of atrophy of the muscles and ankylosis of the involved joint.

3. Anatomy of the vertebral column

To understand the neuraxial anatomy it is necessary to develop a concept of the relationship between surface and bony anatomy pertinent o the neuraxial structures. The vertebral column is formed by the superposition of the 33 vertebrae that stand from the occipital to the sacrum and coccyx. Each vertebra is formed by a body in the anterior aspect and a ring in its posterior region. From each ring, except from the first one, appendixes are given off to the sides and posteriorly. One over the other produces the vertebral column and the posterior arches form a tube with lateral holes, from which the nerves leave the spinal canal where the spinal cord resides.

Surrounding the spinal cord in the bony vertebral column are three membranes: the pia mater, the arachnoid mater, and the dura mater. The pia mater is a highly vascular membrane that closely invests the spinal cord. The arachnoid mater, nonvascular membrane that is closely attached to the outermost layer, the dura mater. Between the pia mater and the arachnoid mater is the space of interest in spinal anesthesia, the subarachnoid space. In this space are the CSF, spinal nerves, a trabecular network between the two membranes, blood vessels that supply the spinal cord, and the lateral extensions of the pia mater, the dentate ligaments. In the adult, the lower extent of the spinal cord, the conus medullaris, ends approximately at L1. In the infant the conus medullaris may extend until to L_3. To produce a spinal anesthesia the subarachnoid space is reached by a needle that comes from the skin through the intervertebral space between their posterior spines and pierces the dura mater. Confirmation relies on back flow of CSF to permit the injection of the local anesthetic.

4. Incidence

Paresthesia is an abnormal sensation that occurs during the insertion of a spinal, epidural, combined spinal-epidural (CSE) or continuous spinal needle, a reported frequency ranging from 6.3% to 20% [4-6,8]. It is a widespread assumption that needle-induced paresthesia could be produced by contact of the tip of the needle with a spinal nerve root in the epidural space or with a spinal nerve within the intervertebral foramen. Various factors may influence the occurrence of paresthesia, including the needle-tip configuration, the use of needle-through-needle CSE technique versus single-shot spinal technique, the use of CSE kits with longer spinal needles, or the technique of puncture.

Serious neurologic complication is a rare event. Among the lesions, very little has been written on persistent paresthesia or motor inability. Paresthesia occurred during lumbar spinal block is very frequent in our everyday practice. The nerves, derived from the union of the sensitive and motor roots of the spinal cord are independent structures that macroscopically have their origin in the union of the posterior and anterior rootlets that emerge from the spinal cord in the posterolateral sulcus (sensitive rootlets) and from the anterolateral sulcus (motor rootlets). Each species travel to the intervertebral foramina where anterior and posterior rootlets unite to form a motor root and a sensitive root before joining together to emerge the spinal canal as a nerve. Motor rootlets (anterior) and sensitive rootlets (posterior) occupy the central axis of the spinal canal from the conus medullaris downward.

During the lumbar puncture, the needle is introduced in the dural sac and enters a short distance where there is no nerve rootlets. If the needle goes further, it will make contact with the nerve rootlets that occupy the posterior zone and central posterior zone of the dural sac. Paresthesia would be originated from central zone if the lumbar space was approached sagittally. Or from more lateral rootlets if the needle is deviated from the sagittal plane.

5. Approaching the subarachnoid space

5.1 Position

During lumbar puncture, the position of the patient and adequate flexion of the lumbar backbone must be searched. It will open the space between the vertebrae and will facilitate the approach of the spinal needle to the dural sac, avoiding its contact with the bones. Spinal puncture is carried out in three positions: lateral decubitus, sitting position and jackknife prone position. In both the lateral decubitus and sitting positions, the use of a well-trained assistant is essential if the block is to be easily administered by anesthesiologist in a time-efficient manner. In some patient, the sitting position can facilitate location of the midline, especially in obese patients.

The position of the patient during lumbar puncture may influence the incidence of paresthesia. The incidence of paresthesia is more probable when blocks are preformed with the patient in the lateral position, because of inadvertent spine rotation [10].

5.2 Level

Spinal anesthesia is unparalleled in the way a small mass of drug, virtually devoid of systemic pharmacologic effect, can produce profound, reproducible surgical anesthesia. Spinal anesthesia can be performed at any level of the spine, depending on what the anesthesiologist wants or what the patient needs. Most of the spinals are made in the lumbar interspaces of L_3-L_4 or L_4-L_5, through the puncture of the dura/arachnoid mater, which is deliberately done [3,4].

5.3 Needle

One of the first decisions to be made in considering spinal puncture is what kind of needle to use. For spinal needles there are two main categories: those that cut the dura mater and those that spread the dural fibers. The former include the traditional disposable spinal needle, the Quincke-Babcock needle, and the latter category contains the Greene, Whitacre, and Sprotte needles. The use of small bore needles reduce the incidence of postdural puncture headache. Theoretically, Sprotte needles should present a higher index of paresthesia than the Quincke needles. But this theory has not been proved, and there are many papers that state the same incidence.

5.4 Paramedian or median access

It was not found in the literature any study comparing the incidence of paresthesia with the use of the paramedian *vs* median approach of the spinal canal.

5.5 Combined spinal-epidural

The combined spinal-epidural (CSE) technique is designed to combine the advantages of spinal and epidural anesthesia. Spinal anesthesia can offer a rapid complete conduction block, and epidural anesthesia using an epidural catheter can easily prolong anesthetic duration and may be used to provide postoperative analgesia. CSE anesthesia was first performed using the double segment technique [11]. However, the needle-through-needle technique has gained popularity [12]. In terms of spinal needle insertion, paresthesia frequency was more than twice as high for the needle-through-needle group than for the double segment technique group, although we were not able to establish a statistical difference between the two techniques [13]. According to others authors, the frequency of paresthesia was 9% for single-shot spinal anesthesia and 37% during spinal needle insertion of needle-through-needle, which was significant [14]. One possible reason for the higher frequency of paresthesia during spinal needle insertion in the needle-through-needle was the length of spinal needles introduced into the subarachnoid space. A spinal needle guided by an epidural needle rarely meets tissue resistance until it reaches the dura mater, and thus the dura mater is easily and deeply perforated [15,16].

The majority of these papers were observed in obstetric patients. Comparing single shot spinal anesthesia, combined spinal-epidural blocks and continuous spinal anesthesia in orthopedic surgery of elderly patients no significant difference was observed among population [17].

5.6 The use of the introducer

During lumbar puncture, the interaction of the needle and the tissue may produce a deflection of the needle tip. This deflection of the needle may increase the incidence of paresthesia. The use of introducers reduce the deflection of the needles [18,19]. The deflection is greater with beveled needles as compared to the pencil point needles, and also greater when using thinner needles as compared to the larger bore needles. In the single shot subarachnoid technique, removing the stylet when the needle tip still is in the interspinous ligament plus a continuous forward movement until CSF is drained may reduce the incidence of paresthesia [10].

6. Conclusion

Paresthesia during regional anesthesia increases patient discomfort and the risk of abrupt movement but, more importantly, paresthesia may be associated with neurological damage.

A large prospective study conducted in France reported that nerve injury is rare, but that it is often associated with paresthesia during the administration of a block or pain on injection [9]. Compared to non-paresthesia patients, long-term neurological sequela have been reported more frequently in patients that have experienced paresthesia during regional anesthesia [6]. Direct trauma to nerve roots or the spinal cord may manifest as paresthesia. When transient paresthesias occur during spinal needle placement it is appropriate to stop and assess for the presence of CSF in the needle hub, rather than withdraw and redirect the spinal needle away from the side of paresthesia as some authors have suggested.

7. References

[1] Lee RA, van Zundert AAJ, Breedveld P, Wondergem JHM, Peek D, Wieringa PA. The anatomy of the thoracic spinal canal investigated with magnetic resonance imaging (MRI). Acta Anaesth Belg 2007;58:163-167.

[2] Imbelloni LE, Quirici MB, Ferraz-Filho JR, Cordeiro JA, Ganem EM. The anatomy of the thoracic spinal canal investigated with magnetic resonance imaging. Anesth Analg 2010;110:1494-1495.

[3] van Zundert AAJ, Stultiens G, Jakimowicz JJ, Peek D, van der Hamk WGJM, Korsten HHM, Wildsmith JAW. Laparoscopic cholecystectomy under segmental thoracic spinal anaesthesia: a feasibility study. Br J Anaesth 2007;98:682-686.

[4] Imbelloni LE, Pitombo PF, Ganem EM. The incidence of paresthesia and neurologic complications after lower spinal thoracic puncture with cut needle compared to pencil point needle. Study in 300 patients. J Anesth Clinic Res 2010;1:106 - Open Access www.omicsonline.org - doi:10.4172/2155-6148.1000106.

[5] Auroy Y, Benhamou D, Bargues L, Ecoffey C. Falissard B, Mercier FJ, Bouaziz H, Samii K. Major complications of regional anesthesia in France. The SOS regional anesthesia hotline service. Anesthesiology 2002;97:1274-1280.

[6] Horlocker TT, McGregor DG, Matsushige DK, Schroeder DR, Besse JA. A retrospective review of 4767 consecutive spinal anesthetics: central nervous system complications. Perioperative outcomes group. Anesth Analg 1997;84:578-584.

[7] Pong RP, Gmelch BS, Bernards CM. Does a paresthesia during spinal needle insertion indicate intrathecal needle placement? Reg Anesth Pain Med 2009;34:29-32.

[8] Tetzlaff JE, Dilger JA, Wu C, Smith MP, Bell G. Influence of lumbar spine pathology on the incidence of paresthesia during spinal anesthesia. Reg Anesth Pain Med 1998;23:560-563.

[9] Auroy Y, Narchi P, Messiah A, Litt L, Rouvier B, Samii K. Serious complications related to regional anesthesia: results of a prospective survey in France. Anesthesthesiology 1997:87:479-486.

[10] Palacio Abizanda FJ, Reina MA, Fornet I, López A, López López MA, Morillas Sendín P. Parestesias y anestesia subaracnóidea en cesáreas: estúdio comparativo según la posición de la paciente. Rev Esp Anestesiol Reanim 2009;56:21-26.

[11] Brownridge P. Epidural and subarachnoidal analgesia for elective caesarean section (letter). Anaesthesia, 1981; 36:70.

[12] Coates MB. Combined subarachnoid and epidural techniques (letter). Anaesthesia, 1982; 37:89-90.

[13] Ahn HJ, Choi DH, Kim CS. Paraesthesia during the needle-through-needle and the double segment technique for combined spinal epidural anaesthesia. Anaesthesia 2006;61:634-638.

[14] McAndrew CR, Harms P. Paraesthesiae during needle-through-needle combined spinal epidural versus single-shot spinal elective caesarean section. Anaesth Intens Care 2003;31:514-517.

[15] Lyons G, MacDonald R, Mikl B. Combined epidural/spinal anaesthesia for caesarean section. Through the needle or in separates spaces? Anaesthesia 1992;47:199-201.

[16] Browne IM, Birnbach DJ, Stein DJ, O'Gorman DA, Kuroda M. A comparison of Espocan and Tuohy needles for the combined spinal-epidural technique for labor analgesia. Anesth Analg 2005;101;535-540.

[17] Imbelloni LE, Beato L. Comparação entre raquianestesia, bloqueio combinado raqui-peridural e raquianestesia contínua para cirurgias de quadril em pacientes idosos. Estudo retrospectivo. Rev Bras Anestesiol 2002;52:316-325.

[18] Ahn WS, Bhk HH, Lim Yj, Kim YC. The effect of introducer gauge, design and bevel direction on the deflection of spinal needles. Anaesthesia 2002;57:1007-1011.

[19] Sitzman BT, Uncles DR. The effects of needle type, gauge, and tip bend on spinal needle deflection. Anesth Analg 1996;82:297-301.

5

Paresthesias as Reflection of the Lateral Asymmetry of Neural Function in Human

Olex-Zarychta Dorota
Academy of Physical Education in Katowice
Poland

1. Introduction

1.1 Neural asymmetry in human - An overview

Most biological systems demonstrate some degree of asymmetry. From lower animals to human normal variation and specialization produce asymmetries of both function and structure. The term asymmetry is often substituted for the term laterality and indicate left-right differences, especially in neurosciences and psychology (Bryden, 1982). However, researchers generally use the term asymmetry in more global context of both structural and functional side dissimilarities while the term laterality is typically used exclusively in relation to functional asymmetry (Hughdahl, 2005). In numerous species representing major vertebrate taxa asymmetries of brain and behaviour have been demonstrated and it is supposed to be an universal feature of the vertebrate nervous system (Goutiérrez-Ibañez et al., 2011; Tommasi, 2009). In a neuroscience perspective the concepts of asymmetry in humans are closely tied to the two hemispheres of the brain (Grabowska et al., 1994; Hughdahl, 2005). Despite the mirror symmetrical organization of the body along the vertical body axis, the two brain hemispheres differ in their anatomy and function; moreover, asymmetries in the brain's functional layout and cytoarchitecture have been correlated with asymmetrical behavioural traits - handedness, footedness, auditory perception, motor preferences and also sensory acuity (see Toga & Thompson, 2003 for review). Studies on anatomical asymmetries in the brain showed differences in distribution of tissue between hemispheres, although they are similar in both weight and volume (Toga & Thompson, 2003). Structural and neurochemical asymmetries in the majority of studies were reported to be linked with functional asymmetries of the brain and behaviour (especially the handedness). Some research showed cytoarchitectural asymmetry in the *planum temporale* related to handedness- marked leftward volume asymmetry. Additionally, this was also related to the degree of right-handedness of participants (Habib et al., 1995). In experiments with MRI Steinmetz observed greater asymmetry of this structure in right-handers in comparison to left-handers (Steinmetz, 1996). Structural asymmetry of central sulcus was reported to fit with the functional hemispheric asymmetry in relation to handedness (Babiloni et al., 2003), what indirectly confirms the relationship of laterality pattern in limbs and the motor cortex structure and function. Some investigators found differences between two brain hemispheres in levels of neurotransmitters (dopamine, norepinephrine), what was linked with various behavioural asymmetries (Glick, Ross & Hough 1982; Tucker &

Williamson, 1984). Generally, asymmetry in the neuromotor performance is assumed to be linked with the brain functional and laterality i.e. hemispheres specialization (Springer & Deutsch, 2004; Tommasi, 2009). Functional asymmetry of the human brain is related to different behavioural traits. One of the earliest observations of brain asymmetry was the specialization of the left hemisphere for language functions (Binder, 2000). Some research has pointed towards the right hemisphere as being specialized for spatial processing and emotional control (Springer & Deutsch, 2004) and all this came to develop standard models of hemispheric asymmetry claiming that each hemisphere has its own characteristic domain of competence - the left hemisphere is commonly regarded as the verbal and logical brain area, the right hemisphere is responsible for creativity and spatial relations. However, brain function lateralization is evident in the phenomena of right- or left-handedness and of right or left ear preference, but a person's preferred hand is not a clear indication of the location of brain function. Although 95% of right-handed people have left-hemisphere dominance for language, only 18.8% of left-handed people have right-hemisphere dominance for language function. Additionally, 19.8% of the left-handed present bilateral language functions (Springer & Deutsch, 2004). All these findings seem to link the neural asymmetry with motor and sensory traits in human. More recent studies confirmed asymmetry as the norm when the it comes to functions of he brain and nervous system, however researchers underline the fact that lateralization of the brain functions varies depending on several individual biological and environmental factors and also their interactions (Grabowska et al., 1994; Olex-Zarychta & Raczek, 2008; Tommasi, 2009). Manifestation of lateralization of the brain and nervous system can be explicitly observed in handedness as well as in footedness, which expresses in consistent preference for one arm or leg over the other in certain motor tasks. Therefore handedness and footedness in human has been linked with the asymmetry of the motor control system.

1.2 Laterality and motor control

Studies on human motor control incorporate research on different types of movements. Generally, movements can be graded along the scale from the most to the least automatic. It has been suggested that different neurophysiologic processes are involved in phylogenetically old behaviors like reflex reactions or rhythmic patterned outputs and discrete movements like grasping or reaching (Rothwell, 1996; Schaal et al., 2004). Lateral asymmetry is a prominent, but still poorly understood aspect of the human motor performance in all mentioned above types of movements. Lateralization of motor performance emphasized by handedness and footedness is characterized by the consistent preference for one extremity over the other in performing the majority of motor actions (Bagesteiro & Sainburg, 2002, 2003). Generally, it is accepted that handedness and footedness results from different (i.e. lateralized) neural control of each extremity with an assumption that motor asymmetry is a feature of neural organization of motor control (Shabbott & Sainburg, 2008; Wang & Sainburg, 2007). Although a feature of arm and leg preferences is well-documented in humans and nonhuman primates (Hopkins & Pearson 2000; Hopkins et al. 2003) there is still a lot of disagreement concerning the emergence of this phenomena. Lateral differences in motor performance have been reported in many tasks requiring speed, accuracy, and fast reaction time, typically with the better results for the dominant extremity (Annett, 1992; Elliott & Heath, 1999; Hore et. al. 1998; Olex- Zarychta & Raczek, 2008; Peters 1991). Differences in neural mechanisms of movement control among different laterality patterns have been suggested with emphasis to the not exclusively central, but also peripheral control to be involved (Aziz-Zadeh et.al., 2006; Kato & Asami, 1998; Olex, 2004; Olex-Zarychta et.al. 2009). One of the first studies on handedness was published by Liepmann (1905) who suggested that the hemisphere which is contralateral to the dominant arm is as well dominant. As such it plans movements of both arms. Since that time considerable body of evidence has confirmed the hypothesis that cerebral hemisphere contralateral to the dominant arm plays a particular role in the performance of both arms. Several studies suggested that this hemisphere (hereafter referred to as the "dominant hemisphere") and premotor areas are more active comparing to the nondominant equivalent during ipsilateral (Kim et al. 1993; Kawashima et al., 1997), contralateral (Kim et al. 1993; Dassonville et al. 1997; Taniguchi, 1999) and bilateral arm movements (Kim et al., 1993). Additionally, brain damage subject studies with unilateral lesions have revealed movement deficits in the non-dominant arm when the dominant hemisphere was damaged, but not in the dominant arm movement after lesions to the non-dominant hemisphere (Haaland & Harrington, 1994, 1996). This suggests that the dominant hemisphere encloses special circuitry for the control of both arms. Reflection of Liepmann's model of motor lateralization can be seen in the hypothesis that dominant arm advantages in performance exist due to specialization of the dominant hemisphere for the visual-mediated correction processes (Carson et al., 1990). Several studies supported this hypothesis and indicated that dominant arm movements tend to be shorter in duration (Elliot, 1993; Mieschke et al., 2001; Todor & Cisneros 1985) and more accurate (Roy, 1983; Todor & Cisneros, 1985) than non-dominant arm movements. Additionally, based on findings made by Flowers (1975) one can hypothesize that interlimb differences in movement accuracy tend to be reduced when movements are performed at high velocity, which elicit decrease of the role of visual-based error corrections. This way, feedback correction model of the lateralization predicts that the dominant arm should show distinct advantages in the timing and efficacy of corrections to visual errors. There is alternative explanation of the dominant arm advantages during reaching introduced by Sainburg (2002, 2005). It was named by the author "the dynamic dominance hypothesis" of motor lateralization and is based on the idea that a movement is initially planned by specifying trajectory parameters in an extrapersonal space (Sarlegna & Sainburg, 2007). This plan is transformed into commands that specify the dynamic properties that reflect the forces required to initiate the movement (Sainburg, 2002). This hypothesis suggests specialization of the dominant arm control in a process of dynamic transformations. Further research lead to the hypothesis that the nondominant arm controller has become specialized for regulating limb impedance, which is needed to achieve steady-state positions (Bagesteiro & Sainburg, 2003, 2005; Duff and Sainburg, 2006; Schabowsky et al., 2007). Footedness has been previously reported as an important factor in predicting the motor preparation dependent on the behavioural context of a particular task (Carpes et al., 2007; Gabbard & Iteya, 1996; Grouios et al., 2009). It has been claimed that the footedness may be a better predictor of the cerebral lateralization than the handedness (Elias, Bryden & Bulman-Fleming, 1998; Elias & Bryden, 1998; Strauss & Wada, 1983). This seems to confirm the important role of the laterality both upper and lower extremities in detecting the asymmetry of the neural organization in human. It was suggested that motor performance of upper limbs is influenced only by the central information processing, while the effect for lower limbs is influenced by the peripheral motor control (Kato & Asami, 1998). However, some other findings strongly suggested the role of peripheral factors in rapid movements performed with hands what partly contradict models and theories based on hands performance asymmetries as an effect of exclusively central motor control (Jaric, 2000). In neurophysiologic studies it was hypothesized that the motor laterality may reflect differentially lateralized activation in the motor control system influenced by a central information processing (hemispheric specialization) and also by other structures and processes on levels of motor control such as locomotor's centers of limbs performance (CPGs) and spinal cord (Francis & Spiriduso, 2000; Schaal, 2004; Aziz-Zadeh et al., 2006; Knikou, 2007; Olex-Zarychta & Raczek, 2008; Zehr et al., 2004, 2007). All these findings suggest the neural plasticity to be involved in the motor control system in human. The term of neural plasticity was introduced for the first time by polish neuroscientist Jerzy Konorski in middle XX century (see Zieliński, 2006 for review). According to the theory of neuroplasticity learning and training actually may change both the brains's anatomy and functional organization from top to bottom. It suggests that the pattern of a neuronal activation in CNS changes in response to experience. The concept of neuroplasticity is associated with an experience-driven alteration of synaptic structure and functions: the long-term potentation (LTP) in hippocampus and motor cortex and the long-term depression (LTD) especially in cerebellum, what must influence the process of the motor control (Rothwell, 1996; Monfils et. al., 2005; Aagard et.al., 2002; Agaard, 2003; Fazeli & Collingridge, 1996). Experience-dependent plasticity and asymmetric behaviours may therefore induce different neuronal changes in the motor cortex of the two hemispheres. In interesting experiments on animals (rats and mice) asymmetric use of paws resulted in changes in cell packing density in the motor cortex, and limb preference was related to the asymmetry of sensory input (Diaz, Pinto-Hamuy & Fernandez, 1994). Therefore, it is possible that the lateral asymmetry in motor performance may result from a lateralized sensory stimulation in human development.

1.3 Neural asymmetry studies with the use of the spinal circuit research

Although the simplicity of psychomotor tests makes them an attractive means of assessing motor laterality, a neurophysiologic examination of motor and sensory functions of peripheral nerves seems to be necessary in such investigation (Goble, 2007). In motor control research extensively used tools to study the neural control of movement and to gain detailed understanding of the nervous system plasticity are the motor evoked potential techniques, with a special emphasis to the spinal reflexes circuits. Despite the detail neural mechanisms involved in motor control are still unknown, the multidimensional and temporal regulation of limb mechanics by spinal circuits is assumed to be attached to neural proprioreceptive feedback from muscles and sensory receptors as well as to organization of descending command and motor output from the spinal cord. (Christou et al., 2002; Kimura, 2001; Rothwell, 1996; Zehr 2002, 2004; Zehr & Wolpaw, 2006; Misiaszek, 2003; Olex-Zarychta et al., 2009; Olex-Zarychta, 2010). One of the most extensively studied reflexes in the literature on human neurophysiology is a Hoffmann reflex (H-reflex). The relative ease with which this reflex can be elicited in muscles throughout the human body and few neural parameters involved in this circuit makes it a very attractive research tool in motor control research (Misiaszek, 2003; Zehr & Wolpaw, 2006). Studies incorporating the H-reflex as a neural probe showed changes in excitability of the reflex occur while movement actions and also in the absence of movement what suggests the existence of intrinsic modulating factors in motor control system, connected with the spinal circuit organization and/or with transmission parameters in motor and sensory pathways (Aymard et al, 2000; Kimura, 2001;

Misiaszek, 2003; Zehr et. al, 2004; Zehr, 2006; Zehr et.al., 2007). Previous studies with the H–reflex demonstrated clearly that adaptive plasticity could be induced in the spinal cord and that it could be examined by using the H-reflex (Agaard, 2003; Carp & Wolpaw, 1994; Wolpaw & Chen, 2006). Some researchers have investigated the effectiveness of the Ia monosynaptic pathway in leg muscles in relation to the handedness. Goode et al. (1980) observed a lateralization of the H-reflex responsiveness towards the non-dominant side, which was significant only in case of right-handed participants. Other findings showed the recovery curve lateralization of the H-reflex from the wrist flexors (Tan, 1989). The amplitude of the H-reflex was shown to depend on muscle use and exercise, what suggests the possible relation of the laterality and the plasticity of neural pathways (Mynark & Koceja, 1997; Sigh & Maini, 1980). Previous studies from our laboratory indicated significant depression of the H-reflex on dominant side in groups of both left-sided (left-handed/ left-footed) and right-sided participants (Olex-Zarychta et. al., 2008), what suggests that this effect may be associated with greater central steering influences on the dominant side in confirmation of previous findings that depression of the H-reflex is the dominant corticospinal effect on interneurones projecting the Ia afferents (Aymard et al., 2000). Previous results showed also differences in a sensory (Vs) and motor (Vm) conduction velocity between two examined laterality patterns. Higher values of the Vs in the non-dominant extremity in right-sided participants were recorded, what may contribute to a relatively better perception by the right cerebral hemisphere in this group of subjects. A lack of such effect in left-sided participants was interpreted as an effect of more symmetrical motor activity related to the right-sided social pressures in daily life or/and of a possible different pattern of the cerebral perception in this group of subjects (Olex-Zarychta et. al., 2008; Olex-Zarychta 2010). The selective hemispheric activation may thus play a role in the motor output asymmetry in human extremities. Assuming that the afferent sensory feedback is the neural basis for interlimb coordination and contributes strongly to the modulation of the spinal reflexes as well as control on supraspinal levels (Freitas et al., 2007; Pearson and Gordon, 2000; Rothwell, 1996; Zehr et al., 2004; Zehr, 2006), it was hypothesized that the functional dominance in limbs may be an important modulating factor for the motor coordination (Olex-Zarychta & Raczek, 2008; Olex-Zarychta, 2010). Earlier studies indicated asymmetries in the number of corticospinal axons (Nathan et al., 1990) as well as in cortical representations of the dominant limb muscles (Nudo, 1992) and brought evidences supporting the adaptive plasticity in muscle and cutaneous afferent reflex pathways induced by training and rehabilitative interventions. The activity-dependent plasticity of the neural system was found in both strength and endurance training (Olmo et. al., 2006). Changes of the H-reflex amplitude were found in the trained leg after couple of weeks of heavy strength training, with no such effect in untrained leg despite the comparable gains in strength due to cross - education program (Zehr, 2006) The increase of the H-reflex response was observed during maximal muscle contraction after resistance training (Aagard et al., 2003). Authors suggested the existence of chronic plastic adaptations in the Ia spinal reflex pathway leading to increased reflex excitability and co-existence of both spinal and supraspinal contributions to reflexes due to external factors. The existence of neural adaptation mechanisms has been suggested to comprise an increased central motor drive, elevated motoneuron excitability and changes in a presynaptic inhibition (Aagard, 2002). The motor laterality research brought some evidence that laterality pattern in limbs is related to the lateralization of excitability in the motor system, connected with interhemispheric inhibition as a function of handedness (Baümer et al., 2007). All these findings enabled to suppose that laterality pattern may strongly influence the motor control process and neural asymmetry (Marchand-Pauvert et al., 1999; Olex-Zarychta & Raczek, 2008). However, in the majority of cited interesting experiments the model of laterality pattern in hand-foot combination was not provided. When the handedness of participants was taken into consideration, results of bilateral studies confirmed differences in lateral asymmetries of the H-reflex in right and left handed participants (Goode et al., 1980). Other experiments with respect of the sidedness of participants (preference of hand and foot on the same body side) indicated significant depression of the soleus H-reflex amplitude in the dominant lower extremity in those laterality patterns, what strongly suggests that inhibition of the soleus H-reflex on the dominant side what may be related to descending motor commands associated with greater cortical influences on the dominant side (Olex-Zarychta, 2010).

1.3.1 Paresthesias and neural asymmetry in human

The special attention during experiments incorporating the evoked potentials should be paid to the feedback from participants. Cooperation with patient before, during and after the laboratory session is crucial for obtaining proper results of neurophysiologic testing taking into consideration influence of patient-dependent factors as an emotional state, any voluntary movement or even a motivation or attitude towards procedures (Kimura, 2001; Misiaszek 2003; Zehr et al., 2004, 2006, 2007). Before neurophysiologic testing, especially the bilateral one and in healthy participants careful screening of handedness/footedness should be provided, in order to detect any possible factor influencing the asymmetry of future results. At least self-reported handedness/footedness should be recorded, however, sometimes participants are not conscious about their footedness and more specific laterality tests should be recommended (f.ex. footedness test by Chapman, 1987). During testing the special care should be taken to the symmetry protocol to avoid erroneous results. In neurophysiologic testing , the use of feedback monitors during laboratory sessions makes the feedback from participant/patient not decisive or crucial for eliciting the proper results of testing. However, patients always have own feelings about the situation of testing which should not be omitted or underestimated by the researcher or medical staff. Paresthesias, sensations of tingling, pricking, or numbness of skin during surface stimulation of the nerve (electrical or magnetic) are the most common feedback from patient during neurophysiologic testing which have no apparent long-term physical effect and are totally harmless for the patient (Miller, 1986; Olex- Zarychta et al., 2009). Paresthesias are common, transient symptoms of inhibiting or stimulating of the function of the nerve. Removing the pressure from the nerve (i.e. removing the stimulation electrode from the skin) typically results in gradual relief of these sensations. The incidence of paresthesias during electrical stimulation depends on many individual factors related to the body composition, neural system characteristics and also factors attached to experimental conditions (Miller, 1986). Paresthetic sensations are used by anesthesiologists to localization of nerves and target areas in regional anaesthesia procedures as standard technique of needle positioning f.ex. in nerve blocks (Miller, 1986), but transient paresthesias are often underestimated in neurophysiologic testing with the use of the evoked potentials method. Transient asymmetrical paresthesias during sensorimotor testing are common and harmless, and should be more appreciated by physicians and researchers as a valuable information on individual level of the neural asymmetry. Taking into consideration the assumption that asymmetry of the human neural system is a normal, physiological phenomenon (see paragraph 1.1 of this chapter) it seems quite logical that the handedness/footedness should be related to the level of neural reactions on the peripheral level. Therefore, the possibility of the physiologic neural asymmetry should be taken into consideration during both symmetrical or asymmetrical testing with the method of evoked potentials. Neural feedback from the patient - among others also paresthesias - may be therefore a reflection of the neural function on both central and peripheral level of the neural system. Bilateral testing makes a good opportunity for comparison the asymmetry of the neural feedback from the patient during nerve stimulation. Observations of differences between the motor and the sensory feedback from the dominant and the non dominant extremities may bring some additional information about the neural state of the patient and may help in diagnosis. Taking into consideration previous findings on motor control mechanisms it is possible that laterality (limb dominance) is related to structural asymmetry of the neural system, what may influence a conduction process in peripheral nerves. Asymmetrical paresthesias are typical in some demyelination disorders as sclerosis multiplex (SM) and indicate hyperexcitability of demyelinated axons, however there is no specific data on relations of the handendness/footedness and a pattern of paresthesias in SM and other demyelination diseases patients. There is also no reference data of the neural asymmetry in healthy population–some authors indicate 5% as a normal asymmetry range in neurophysiologic testing, however in sport physiology and rehabilitation side differences in healthy participants exceed sometimes 40% as the effect of the asymmetrical muscle stimulation in sport training or daily life (Olmo et al., 2006; Shewmann, 2007). All this suggests that the neural asymmetry should be treated as a normal, physiological phenomenon and probably depends on learning, experience and personal activity model of the person with the special role of a physical activity history. Asymmetrical paresthesias during the neurophysiologic testing both in health and disease may be thus related (at least partially) to the physiologic neural asymmetry. It may be sometimes a helpful diagnostic hint for researchers and medical staff. In the light of all mentioned above, side asymmetries in results of any neurophysiologic testing do not necessarily indicate a pathological process in human and caution should be exercised in interpreting lateral asymmetries of results. The knowledge of the normal function of the peripheral nervous system is important to physicians. Only by understanding of normal recordings may proper diagnoses be achieved. Described below results of a simple experiment incorporating the H-reflex elicited in healthy young adults may be the contribution for detecting the role of careful handedness/footedness screening before neurophysiologic testing and the role of paresthesias as a reflection of the neural asymmetry in human.

2. Lateral differences in neurophysiologic testing: The H-reflex study on healthy adults

2.1 Aim of research

The aim of this experiment was to investigate the effect of the laterality pattern in limbs on the H-reflex asymmetry in groups of participants with four laterality patterns in hand-foot combination: two congruent and two crossed ones. Analysis of asymmetries in sensory and/or motor parameters of the spinal circuits among experimental groups are expected to throw a new light on the effect of the laterality pattern on the motor control system in human. Taking into consideration mentioned earlier findings on the human laterality, individuals with crossed patterns in the hand–foot combination are expected to present different level of the neural asymmetry than congruent ones. Paresthesias are expected to be valuable indicators of the neural asymmetry and are also expected to be attached to the laterality pattern (footedness and/or handedness) of participants. Differences in sensory or/and motor parameters of the spinal circuit among experimental groups would throw a new light on the effect of the laterality pattern in limbs on plasticity of motor control system in human. Results are expected to contribute introduced before hypothesis (Olex-Zarychta & Raczek, 2008; Olex-Zarychta, 2010) that the functional dominance of human limbs is an important modulating factor in the motor control system in human. According to this hypothesis asymmetry of the motor performance may be an evidence for the behavior-induced plasticity of the CNS. Thus, the motor asymmetry may be an effect of the integration process of information from both ascending and descending neural pathways. Moreover, the limb dominance may be an effect of the cortical re-mapping and may influence the function of the whole motor control system, with an assumption that greater central steering influences should affect the dominant (more experienced) side. Asymmetrical paresthesias during neurophysiologic testing may be therefore a reflection of structural/ functional differences in the nervous system, what was previously supposed as a result of training and experience (Zehr, 2006). Therefore, the pattern of paresthesias during testing is expected to fit the pattern of the handedness/footedness of participants. Results of an experiment incorporating the H-reflex are expected to throw a new light on relations between the laterality and the neural asymmetry in human.

2.2 Participants

A total of 33 healthy male volunteers aged 21-23 (mean age 21.6, mean height 186±6) participated in a study. The study was accepted by the local Ethics Committee and each participant gave informed consent. Participants were carefully screened to eliminate any current or past neurological or muscle diseases or trauma. The functional dominance of upper and lower extremities of each participant was established by the use of a questionnaire (selection from Edinburgh Handedness Inventory by Oldfield, (1971). Additional items on foot preference were provided according to 11-item foot performance inventory of Chapman that has previously shown good internal consistency and test-retest reliability (Chapman et al., 1987). Self-reported handedness and footedness have also been recorded. Participants qualified for the experiment presented no signs of an ambidexterity both in upper and lower extremities and presented four main laterality patterns in hand-foot combinations. Research group consisted of four subgroups of 10 right-handed and right-footed (RH/RF), 7 right-handed and left-footed (RH/LF), 10 left-handed and left-footed (LH/LF) and 6 left-handed and right-footed (LH/RF) participants.

2.3 Experimental setup and procedures

The soleus H-reflex was elicited in the left and right lower extremity in the same laboratory session for each participant (Brinkworth et al., 2007). All experimental sessions were organized in the same lab with a stable air temperature of 22°C, always in the morning (10-12 AM) to provide the most comparative conditions of an experimental environment for all

participants. (Kimura, 2001; Waxman, 2004). During recording session participants were lying comfortably on stomach, with their head positioned centrally and arms close to the body. No moves were allowed during experiment to prevent any influence on results. The control of the level of alpha motor neuron pool excitability by maintaining bilaterally relaxed soleus muscles during recording session was provided. The position of participants was comfortable for releasing antagonist muscles (tibialis anterior). Monopolar recording Ag/AgCl self adhesive electrode (Sorimex, Poland, diameter 30 mm) was fixed on the soleus muscle distal to the belly of gastrocnemius, medial to the Achilles tendon (Zehr, 2002), symmetrically on the left and right lower extremity, with the use of anatomical landmarks to keep the symmetry. The reference electrode on each leg was localized on patella. To provide a total safety to participants the stimulator was double isolated from a patient by the use of a passive isolation unit (IST-1, Medicor, Hungary) and an additional ground electrode was placed above a recording site. Skin was prepared before by shaving and cleaning with an alcohol swab. The bipolar surface electrode and ST-3 electro stimulator (Medicor, Hungary) were used for stimulating the tibial nerve in the popliteal fossa of each extremity. The non dominant extremity was tested first in all participants, taking into consideration results of previous research indicating greater responsiveness of the H-reflex towards the non-dominant side (Goode et al.,1980). Before recordings some training pulses were provided on each extremity to find the best possible muscle response in the target area, taking into consideration the possibility of morphological differences in the tibial nerve location. The best impact to the nerve was found in each participant by slightly changing the stimulating electrode location in popliteal fossa to obtain the largest electric field in the nerve area. The single square impulses of 0.5 ms duration were triggered from a computer.
Stimuli were applied 10 seconds apart to reduce any effect of a post activation depression of the reflex (Palmieri et al., 2004). Stimulus intensity required to obtain the maximum H-reflex amplitude was determined by increasing the stimulus intensity from 0 in small increments. The stimulus intensity was fixed individually for each participant in a manner to obtain the maximum reflex amplitude in the extremity. Before recordings full H/M recruitment curves (from a stimulus intensity smaller than required to elicit a H-reflex to a stimulus intensity larger than required to reach the maximal M-wave) in both legs were performed to control the experimental setting (Hultborn et al., 1987). On the basis of the H/M ratio any differences in resistance that may occur at the electrode-skin interface and in the soft tissues, as well as differences in electrode placement were recognized and measures were repeated when necessary. Maximal H-reflex amplitudes reached up 60% of the maximal M-waves in all participants, what stayed in concordance with values referenced for healthy adults (Tucker, Tuncer & Türker, 2005). Electromyography signals (EMG) were recorded by CyberAmp 380 amplifier with AI 405 head stages (Axon Instruments, USA). Signals were amplified and filtered in the range of 10-1000 Hz. Data were collected, stored and analyzed by the Axotape-V2 computer software (Axon Instruments, USA). Ten trials for each extremity were recorded and an average of results obtained from all trials was involved in a statistical analysis (Tucker, Tuncer, & Türker, 2005). The following parameters of evoked potentials were recorded: the onset latency of the M-wave (LatMR, LatML) and of the H-reflex (LatHR, LatHL), amplitude of the H-reflex (AHR, AHL) and duration of the H-reflex (TH). Peak-to-peak amplitudes of the H-reflex were measured for each extremity. Onset latencies were measured as time intervals between stimulus artifact and onset of electrical muscle response (latency of the M-wave) in the range of 5-8 ms after the stimulus artifact

and in the range of 30-45 ms (latency of the H-reflex), with the respect of normal values for healthy young adults (Gupta, 2008; Kimura, 2001;Tucker Tuncer, & Türker, 2005) and taking into consideration subjects' height. Duration of the H response was measured from the initial take off to the final return to the baseline, taking into consideration a biphasic waveform of the H-reflex in soleus muscles (Kimura 2001; Tucker et al., 2005). To calculate the asymmetry size in the H-reflex in subjects and among groups of participants the special protocol was introduced to make measurements the most comparable in the aspects of the asymmetry evaluation. In this study relative differences in parameters for dominant and non-dominant legs were provided by the use of the calculated for each participant symmetry coefficients (SC).

2.4 Data analysis

To make a comparison of data obtained in participants with different laterality patterns reliable enough, the symmetry coefficient (SC) for response parameters was calculated for each participant on the basis of the following equation:

$$SC = (X_D - X_N) / (X_D + X_N)$$

where: SC- the relative difference between two sides

- X_D- value for the dominant extremity
- X_N- value for the non dominant extremity

From the methodological point of view, the use of the SC seems to be valuable in asymmetry evaluation. It enables to compare side differences among groups taking into consideration asymmetries between the dominant and non-dominant extremity of each participant in a particular group. It makes comparisons more powerful and more informative. Statistical analyses were done by the use of Statistica software 9.0 (Statsoft, USA). The basic statistics included arithmetic mean (M) and standard deviation (SD) calculated for each parameter and SC. The pair sequence Wilcoxon's test (T) was used for analysis of differences between dominant and non-dominant extremities of participants in subgroups and the nonparametric Mann-Whitney's test (U) were used for analysis of results obtained from groups of right and left-handers with different dominance in lower extremities. The use of non-parametric measures was justified by recognized lack of symmetry in research groups (on the basis of the Kołmogorov-Smirnoff normality test and a visual inspection of the data). The normality assumption of ANOVA was not met, so the distribution-free tests were used as its equivalents.

2.5 Results

2.5.1 Latency

Tendency towards longer latency was observed in the dominant leg in all laterality patterns. In left-handers significantly longer latency was found in the right leg in left-footed participants in relation to right-footed ones U (293,5) $p=0.002$. However, the greatest differences between the H-reflex latency in the dominant and non-dominant lower extremity was found in the group RH/LF, where results of the T test were significant T (11) $p= 0.004$.

2.5.2 Duration

In the duration of the H-reflex the tendency towards prolonged response was observed in dominant leg in right-handers, but with no statistical effect. In left-handers difference in the degree of TH asymmetry varied significantly between left and right footed subjects (see table 2 for details). However, longer duration of the H-reflex was recorded in the dominant extremities of all participants (see table 1 for details).

2.5.3 Amplitude

Left-handers with crossed laterality pattern presented significant depression of the H-reflex amplitude in the non-dominant lower extremity in comparison to left-sided participants (p= 0.014). In right-handed subjects no footedness effect on the amplitude was found (see tables 1 and 2).

parameters	RIGHT-HANDED			LEFT-HANDED	
	Right footed	Left footed	U	Right footed	Left footed
Lat HR	32.75±2.63	33.11±2.69	ns	**35.68±0.95**	**31.49±7.79**
Lat HL	32.72±2.85	37.59±14.02	ns	34.11±3.93	32.67±3.51
AHR	2.23±2.48	2.69±1.85	ns	**1.02±0.13**	**2.91±1.83**
AHL	2.47±2.10	2.65±1.54	ns	1.96±1.17	3.50±1.29
THR	8.19±2.76	8.55±3.16	ns	9.36±3.92	8.42±3.44
THL	8.04±2.08	9.13±4.01	ns	8.45±3.36	9.47±3.82

Lat-latency; A-amplitude; T - duration; H-H-reflex; R - right lower extremity; L-left lower extremity; U - p value in The Mann-Whitney's non parametric test, p<0.05

Table 1. Data summary (means ± SD)

SC	RIGHT-HANDED			LEFT-HANDED	
	RF	LF	U	RF	LF
RL LatH	-0.0004±0.05	-0.0441±0.08	ns	0.0254±0.05	-0.0174±0.05
RL AH	-0.1415±0.43	0.0661±0.53	ns	-0.0907±0.35	0.1178±0.32
RL TH	0.002±0.15	-0.0176±0.23	ns	**0.0483±0.06**	**-0.0579±0.13**

SC- right-left symmetry coefficient; U - p value in The Mann-Whitney's non parametric test
The negative value of the SC indicates the asymmetry towards the non dominant lower extremity in the particular laterality pattern

Table 2. Right-left asymmetries of the H-reflex in subjects

However, it was observed that the degree of asymmetry was greater in two congruent laterality patterns in comparison to crossed ones and this tendency was opposite to the latency of the H-reflex. In right-handed and right-footed participants decrease of the amplitude of the H-reflex in the dominant lower extremity was very distinct in comparison to other laterality patterns in limbs.

However, in totally right-sided participants amplitude of the H-reflex was greater on the non-dominant side in all cases (figure1).

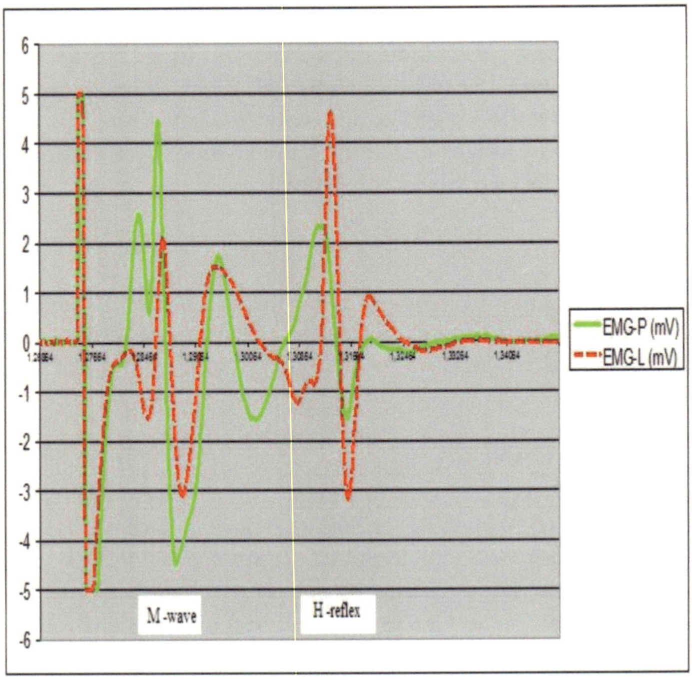

Fig. 1. The electromyographic recording (the averaged data form 10 sweeps) of the right (dominant) and the left lower extremity of participant nr 6 from the group RH/RF. Visible typical for this group depression of the soleus H- reflex in the dominant lower extremity.

Results indicated no particular differences in the side asymmetry degree among laterality patterns in hand-foot combination (see table 1 and 2 for data summaries).

2.5.4 Paresthesias

During experiment right-left differences in feedback from participants were observed. The majority of participants felt tingling in both legs during nerve stimulation and these sensations were not painful or unpleasant for them. In some participants no paresthesias occured (5 persons) or the same levels of sensations on both legs were reported (7). In 1 participant (right-handed and right-footed one) the sensivity on dominant side made recordings of dominant leg difficult (very strong sensations even in very low intensity of impulse was used, with no such problems with testing the left (non-dominant) extremity. Participants reported stronger paresthesias in their dominant extremities in the majority of cases; in this leg minor intensity of electric impulse was needed for eliciting the maximum H-reflex. Stronger sensations during stimulation were attached to the depressed amplitude of the maximum H- reflex. This effect was the most evident in right-handed and right-footed subjects. (figure 1). In this group of participants stronger paresthesias were reported on dominant lower extremity in the majority of tested participants. Left-footed participants generally reported minor side differences in level of paresthesias in comparison to right-footed ones and rarely felt the stimulation discomfortable.

2.6 Discussion

2.6.1 Handedness, footedness and neural asymmetry

Results of this experiment partially confirmed the relationship of the neural asymmetry with the laterality pattern in hand-foot combination and generally indicated relations of asymmetrical paresthesias with results of neurophysiologic testing. Results indicated the laterality pattern in hand-foot combination as a factor influencing somehow reflex pathways probably by an afferent feedback. Footedness influenced the latency and amplitude of the H-reflex especially in left-handed participants, however neural asymmetry seems to be very individual. In previous studies incorporating the H-reflex when only handedness or sidedness of subjects was taken into consideration indicated the statistical effect of the reduced amplitude of the H-reflex in the dominant lower extremity in strongly lateralized, right-handed participants (Goode et al.,1980; Olex-Zarychta, 2010). It was interpreted as an effect of greater central influences on the dominant side, assuming that the normal opposite control is exerted by the motor cortex on primary afferent interneurones in lower and upper limbs. In this experiment the H-reflex amplitude was analyzed in relation to footedness and laterality pattern in hand-foot combination and results were not so obvious- significant effect of footedness occurred only in the left-handed group of subjects. This seems to indicate the footedness to play a greater role in the neural organization in left-handers than right-handers and that not only laterality in the tested extremity, but also laterality pattern in hand-foot combination seems to influence neural asymmetry in human. Neural coupling between upper and lower extremities was previously reported by Knikou (2007), and present results seem to confirm this findings. Recorded differences in H-reflex amplitudes among groups may be associated with laterality-dependent organization of the synaptic transmission as previously suggested (Goode et al., 1980; Olex-Zarychta, 2010). Present results indicate the tendency towards greater side asymmetry in the H-reflex amplitude in two congruent laterality patterns. Taking into consideration that depression of the H-reflex is the dominant corticospinal effect on interneurones projecting the Ia afferents (Aymard et al., 2000) in crossed laterality patterns the cortical effect should be more symmetrical, through the effect on interneurones projecting the Ia afferents from the dominant hand and foot in opposite body sides. According to the neural plasticity concept the muscle use may induce changes in cortical representations of the dominant limb muscles. This makes both left-handed subjects and persons with crossed laterality patterns more complicated in motor functions (Beling, 1998; Olex-Zarychta & Raczek, 2008). Longer duration and longer latency in dominant extremities may indicate the longer central pathway of the reflex in the spinal cord (Rothwell, 1986). Differences in motor and sensory parameters between right and left-handed persons were recorded in some previous studies (Gupta et al., 2008; Tan, 1993). Results may be influenced by strength of limbs' dominance both in upper and lower extremities of participants and they need to be verified in studies on populations selected according to the degree of lateralization in limbs and physical activity models. In this experiment participants were not particularly selected in the aspect of a model of stimulation in their motor activity. Many previous experiments with spinal reflexes suggested multitude factors influence the neural reflex mechanisms in movement and at rest (Goode et al., 1980; Kimura, 2001; Misiaszek, 2003; Sibley et al. 2007; Zehr, 2006). Muscle use is supposed to determine not only the structure of muscles but also the asymmetries in the structure and function of neural pathways (i.e. number of corticospinal axons) and in cortical representations of the dominant limb muscles (Carpes et al., 2007; Fomin & Fomina,

2007; Mynark & Koceja, 1997; Nathan, 1990; Nudo, 1992, Tanaka 2009). In some previous studies asymmetry of the motor units responsiveness did not depend on the biomechanical properties of the muscle tested (Aimonetti et al., 1999). Motor asymmetries thus may contribute to functional differences in rather sensory than motor functions on various levels of the neural system. Present results seem to confirm this suggestion. It was previously suggested that a compound nerve conduction velocity may be a reflection of proprioceptive afferents in human, what corresponds to the neural plasticity concept (Metso et. al., 2008). According to the neural plasticity idea the greater feedback from the dominant side could alter the pattern of neuronal activation in response to experience (Monfils et al., 2005). Previous research brought some evidence for an interhemispheric inhibition as a function of handedness (Baümer et al., 2007). Recorded in this experiment asymmetry of the H-reflex parameters may be thus an effect of different models of motor behaviors that alter the pattern of neuronal activation in human. In this study crossed laterality patterns presented greater side asymmetries than congruent ones in the H–reflex parameters.

2.6.2 Paresthesias as indicators of the neural asymmetry

The pattern of paresthesias observed during testing is similar to previous experiments in our laboratory conducted with the use of the magnetic stimulation (Olex-Zarychta et al., 2009). It suggests the asymmetry of paresthesias to be an effect of the neural system functioning not related to the specific method of testing. Results indicated side differences in paresthesias to be common phenomenon in healthy adults. Stronger sensations on the dominant side observed in participants regardless their handedness (but more evident in right-sided persons) indicate possibility of the existence some structural/functional differences in peripheral nerves related to the laterality and therefore should be taken into consideration in neurophysiologic testing as a valuable information on the nervous system of the patient. Asymmetry of the neural system should be treated as a norm in human and this physiologic asymmetry may influence the result of each neurographic test- presented experiment on healthy young adults indicated a degree of side asymmetries very individual and multidimensional. So, asymmetry of neurography results not always must indicate the pathology or disease, but may be a reflection of the neural asymmetry resulting from experience. Careful screening of the handedness/footedness and a lifestyle model of each patient/participant before any neurophysiologic testing may help achieve the proper diagnosis. The explanation of the mechanism of stronger paresthesias on the dominant side observed during own experiments exceeds the frames of this article and it needs further research. It would be interesting, for example to find out if paresthesias in demyelinating diseases as SM are attached to the handedness/footedness of patients; it would throw a new light to the problem of both origin and treatment of such diseases.

2.7 Conclusion

Results confirmed the concept of neural asymmetry in human as a physiological process, as suggested previously (Tucker & Williamson, 1984). Neural side asymmetry in the H-reflex parameters is probably related to many factors and the laterality pattern in limbs seems to be one of them. Results suggested the laterality pattern in hand-foot combination as a factor influencing the neural plasticity by an afferent feedback. If the hand/foot functional dominance would be an effect of greater amount of experience (motor activity), it may be assumed that this is the factor inducing the changes in neural networks on different stages of motor control by afferent feedback from all extremities. According to the neural plasticity concept the greater feedback from the dominant side could alter behavior by altering the pattern of neuronal activation in response to experience (Monfils et al. 2005). The main conclusion is that the laterality pattern may be a part of a very complicated feedback loop where the motor activity pattern in limbs induces the process of the neural adaptation in response to experience. In the effect both structural and functional changes occur in the motor cortex, what influence the functional organization of the motor control on all levels. This concept may be named the adaptation theory of the motor laterality. Asymmetrical paresthesias during electrophysiologic recordings may be treated as helpful indicators of neural asymmetry in human assuming that the laterality pattern in limbs (handendess and footedness) is a part of a very complicated afferent feedback system where the motor activity is involved in the process of the neural adaptation in response to experience. Asymmetry of motor and sensory reactions of the nervous system, including paresthesias in health and disease may be related to the asymmetry of neural functions in human and these physiologic asymmetries should be taken into consideration in neurophysiologic testing with the use of evoked potentials. If the concept of the neural plasticity related to learning and experience is the proper one, analysis of asymmetry of paresthesias during neurophysiologic testing and other medical procedures might be useful in diagnoses and treatment. They can be a reflection of the complex link between neural and behavioural lateralization in human. This concept needs to be verified on neurophysiologic and behavioral studies on populations with different laterality patterns in hand-foot combinations presenting various models of motor activity; in health and disease.

3. Acknowledgement

The financial support to the project was provided by the Ministry of Science and Higher Education of Poland (grant N 404 045 31/2332).

4. References

Agaard, P. (2003). Training induced changes in neural function. *Exercise and Sport Science Review*, 31, pp. 61-67

Agaard, P., Simonsen, E., Andersen, J., Magnusson, P. & Dyhre-Poulsen, P. (2002). Neural adaptation to resistance training: changes in evoked V-wave and H-reflex responses. *Journal of Applied Physiology*, 92, pp. 2309-2318

Aimonetti, J.M., Morin, D., Schmied, A., Vedel, J.P. & Pagni, S. (1999). Proprioreceptive control of wrist extensor motor units in human: dependence on handedness. *Somatosensory and Motor Research*, 16(1), pp. 11-29

Anett M. (1992). Five tests of hand skill. *Cortex*, 28 pp. 583-600

Aymard, C., Katz, R., Lafitte, C., Lo, E., Penicaud, A., Pradat-Dieh, P. & Raou, S. (2000). Presynaptic inhibition and homosynaptic depression. A comparison between lower and upper limbs in normal human subjects and patients with hemiplegia. *Brain*, 123(8), pp. 1688-1702

Aziz-Zadeh, L., Koski, L., Zaidel, E., Mazziotta, J. & Iacoboni, M. (2006). Lateralization of the human mirror neuron system. *Journal of Neuroscience*, 26(11), pp. 2964-2967

Babiloni, C., Carducci, F., Del Grastta, C., Demartin, M., Romani G. L., Babiloni, F. & Rossini, M. (2003). Hemispherical asymmetry in human SMA during voluntary simple unilateral movements. An fMRI study. *Cortex*, 39, pp. 293-305

Bagesteiro, L. & Sainburg, R. (2002). Handedness: Dominant arm advantages in control of limb dynamics. *Journal of Neurophysiology*, 88, pp. 2408-2421

Bagesteiro, L.B. & Sainburg, R.L. (2003). Nondominant arm advantages in load compensation during rapid elbow joint movements. *Journal of Neurophysiology* 90, pp. 1503–1513

Baümer, T., Dammann, E., Bock, F., Klöppel, S., Siebner, H.R.& Münchau, A. (2007). Laterality of interhemispheric inhibition depends on handedness. *Experimental Brain Research*, 180(2), pp. 195-203

Beling, J., Wolfe, G.A., Allen, K.A. & Boyle, J.M. (1998). Lower extremity preference during gross and fine motor skills performed in sitting and standing postures. *Journal of Orthopedic & Sports Physical Therapy*, 28, pp. 400

Binder, J. (2000). The new neuroanathomy of speech perception. *Brain*. 123(12) ,pp. 2371-2372

Brinkworth, R., Tuncer, M., Tucker, K., Jaberzadech, S. & Türker, K. (2007). Standardization of H-reflex analyses. *Journal of Neuroscience Methods*, 162 (1-2), pp. 1-7

Bryden, M.P. (1982). *Laterality: functional asymmetry in the intact brain*. Academic Press, New York

Carp, J. & Wolpaw, J.R. (1994). Motoneuron plasticity underlying operantly conditioned increase in primate H-reflex. *Journal of Neurophysiology*, 72, pp. 431-442

Carpes F., Rossola, M., Farie, I. & Mota, C. (2007). Influence of exercise intensity on bilateral pedaling symmetry. *Motor Control*, 11 suppl., pp. 39-40

Chapman, J., Chapman, L.& Allen, J. (1987). The measurement of foot preference. *Neuropsychologia*, 25, pp. 597-584

Carson R. G., Chua R., Elliot D. & Goodman D. (1990). The contribution of vision to asymmetries in manual aiming. *Neuropsychologia*. 28, pp. 1215 - 20

Dargent-Pare, C., De Agostini, M., Mesbah, M. & Dellatolas, G. (1992). Foot and eye preferences in adults: Relationship with handedness, sex and age. *Cortex*, 28(3), pp. 343-351.

Dassonville P., Zhu XH., Urgubil K., Kim SG. & Ashe J. (1997). Functional activation in motor cortex reflects the direction and the degree of handedness. *Proceedings of National Academy of Science USA* 94, pp. 14015-14018

Day L.B. & MacNeilage P. F. (1996). Postural asymmetries and language lateralization in humans. *Journal of Comparative Psychology*, 110, pp. 88-98

Diaz, E., Pinto- Hamuy, T. & Fernandez, V. (1994). Interhemispheric structural asymmetry induced by a lateralized reaching task in the rat motor cortex. *European Journal of Neuroscience* 6, pp. 1235-1238

Duff SV, Sainburg R.L. (2006). Lateralization of motor adaptation reveals independence in control of trajectory and steady-state position. Experimental Brain Research 23, pp.156-160

Elias, L.J. & Bryden, M. P. (1998). Footedness is a better predictor of language lateralization than handedness. *Laterality*, 1, pp. 41-51

Elias L.J., Bryden M. P. & Bulman-Fleming M.B. (1998). Footedness is a better predictor than is handedness of emotional lateralization. *Neuropsychologia*, 36, pp. 37-43

Elliott D. (1993). Use of visual feedback during rapid aiming at a moving target. Perceptual and Motor Skills 76 p. 690

Elliot D. & Heath M. (1999). Goal - directed aiming: correcting a force specification error with the right and left hands. *Journal of Motor Behaviour* 31(4), pp. 309-325

Fazeli. R. & Collingridge G. (1996). *Cortical plasticity LTP and LTD*. BIOS Scientific Publishers Ltd, Oxford

Flowers K. (1975). Handedness and controlled movement. *British Journal of Psychology* 66, pp. 39-52

Fomin, R. & Fomina, D. (2007). Presynaptic inhibition of alfa-motoneurones in athletes during different muscular activity. *Motor Control*, 11 suppl., pp. 18-19

Francis, K. & Spiriduso, W. (2000). Age differences in the expression of manual asymmetry. *Experimental Aging Research* 26 (2), pp. 169-181

Freitas, P., Krishnan, V. & Jaric, S. (2007). Force coordination in static manipulation tasks: effect of the change of direction and handedness. *Motor Control* 11 suppl., pp. 114-115

Gabbard, C. & Iteya, M. (1996). Foot laterality in children, adolescents and adults. *Laterality* 1, pp. 199-205

Glick, S.D., Ross, d. A. & Hough, L.B. (1982). Lateral asymmetry of neurotransmitters in human brain. *Brain Research* 234(1), pp. 53-63

Goode, D., Glenn, S., Manning, A. & Middleton, J. (1980). Lateral asymmetry of the Hoffmann reflex: relation to cortical laterality. *Journal of Neurology, Neurosurgery & Psychiatry* 43, pp. 831-835

Goutiérrez-Ibañez C., Reddon A., Kreuzer M.B., Wylie D.R. & Hurd P. (2011). Variation in asymmetry of the habenular nucleus correlates with behavioural asymmetry in cichlid fish. Behavioural Brain Research 221, pp.189-196

Grabowska, A., Herman A., Nowicka A., Szatkowska I. & Szeląg E 91994). Individual differences in the functional asymmetry of the human brain. Acta Neurobiologiae Experimentalis 54, pp. 155-162

Grouios, G., Hatzitaki, V., Kollias, N. & Koidou I. (2009). Investigating the stabilizing and mobilizing features of footedness. *Laterality* 14(4), pp. 362-380

Gupta, N., Sanyal, S., Babbar, R., 2008. Sensory nerve conduction velocity is greater in left handed persons. Indian Journal of Physiology & Pharmacology, 52(2), 189-192

Habib M., Robichon, F., Levrier,O., Khalil R. & Salamon G. (1995). Diverging asymmetries of temporo-parietal cortical areas: a reappraisal of Geschwind/Galaburda theory. Brain Language 48(2), pp. 238-258

Haaland KY. & Harrington DL. (1994). Limb-sequencing deficits after left but not right hemisphere damaged. *Brain and Cognition* 24, pp. 104-122

Haaland, K.Y. & Harrington, D.L. (1996). Hemispheric asymmetries of movement. *Current Opinion in Neurobiology* 6, pp. 796 - 800

Hopkins, W.D., Hook, M., Braccini, S. & Schapiro, S.J. (2003). Population-level right handedness for a coordinated bimanual task in chimpanzees: replication and extension in a second colony of apes. *International Journal of Primatology* 24, pp. 677–689

Hopkins, W.D. & Pearson, K. (2000). Chimpanzee (Pan troglodytes) handedness: variability across multiple measures of hand use. *Journal of Comparative Psychology* 114, pp. 126–135

Hore, J., Watts, S., Tweed, D. & Miller, B. (1998). Overarm throws with the nondominant arm: kinematics and accuracy. *Journal of Neurophysiology* 76 (6), pp. 3693 –3704

Hughdahl, K. (2005). Symmetry and asymmetry in the human brain. European Review 13 supp No 2, pp. 119-133

Hultborn, H., Meunier, S., Morin, C. & Pierrot-Deseilligny, E. (1987). Assessing changes in presynaptic inhibition of Ia fibres: a study in man and cat. *Journal of Physiology* 389, pp. 729-756

Jaric, S. (2000). Is movement symmetry predominantly affected by neural or biomechanical factors?. In: Raczek J, Waskiewicz Z, Juras G, editors. *Current research in motor control*. Katowice: Academy of Physical Education, pp. 37-43

Kato, Y. & Asami, T. (1998). Difference in stimulus - response compatibility effect in premotor and motor time between upper and lower limbs. *Perceptual and Motor Skills* 87, pp. 939 - 946

Kawashima R., Innoue K., Sato K.& Fukuda H. (1997). Functional asymmetry of cortical motor control in left -handed subjects. *Neuroreport* 8, pp. 1729-1732

Kim, S.G., Ashe, J., Hendrich, K., Ellermann, J.M., Merkle, H., Urgubil, K., & Georgopoulos, A.P. (1993). Functional magnetic resonance imaging of motor cortex: hemispheric asymmetry and handedness. *Science* 261, pp. 615-617.

Kimura, J., 2001. *Electrodiagnosis in diseases of nerve and muscle*, 3 rd edition. New York: Oxford University Press

Knikou, M., 2007. Neural coupling between the upper and lower limbs in humans. *Neuroscience Letters*, 416, pp. 138-143

Liepmann, H. (1905). Die linke hemisphäre und das handeln. *Münchener Medizinische Wochenschrift* 49, pp. 2375–2378

Metso, A.J., Palmu, K. & Partanen, J.V. (2008). Compound nerve conduction velocity-a reflection of proprioreceptive afferents? *Clinical Neurophysiology* 119, pp. 29-32

Mieschke, P.E., Elliott, D., Helsen, W.F., Carson, R.G. & Coull, J.A. (2001). Manual asymmetries in the preparation and control of goal-directed movements. *Brain and Cognition* 45, pp. 129–140

Miller, R.D. (Ed.).(1996). *Anaesthesia 2nd edition.* Churchill Livingstone, New York, Edinburgh, London, Melbourne

Misiaszek, J.E. (2003). The H-reflex as a tool in neurophysiology: its limitations and uses in understanding nervous system function. *Muscle & Nerve* 28, pp. 144-160

Monfils, M.H., Bray, D.F., Driscoll ,I., Kleim, J. & Kolb, B. (2005). A quantitative comparison of synoptic density following perfusion versus immersion fixation in the rat cerebral cortex. *Microscopy Research & Technique* 67, pp. 300-304

Mynark, R. & Koceja, D. (1997). Comparison of soleus H-reflex gain from prone to standing in dancers and controls. *Electroencephalography & Clinical Neurophysiology* 105, pp. 135-140

Nardone, A. & Schieppati, M. (1998). Medium-latency response to muscle stretch in human lower limb: estimation of conduction velocity of group II fibres and central delay. *Neuroscience Letters* 249, pp. 29-32

Nathan, P.W., Smith, M.C., & Deacon, P. (1990). The corticospinal tracts in man. *Brain* 113, pp. 303-323

Nudo, R.J., Jenkins, W.M., Merzenich, M.M., Prèjean, T. & Grenda, R. (1992). Neurophysiological correlates of hand preference in primary motor cortex of adult squirrel monkeys. *Journal of Neuroscience* 12, pp. 2918-2947

Ohgaki, K., Nakano, K., Shigeta, H., Kitagawa, Y., Nakamura, N., Iwamoto, K., Makino, M., Takanashi, Y., Kajyama, S. & Kondo, M. (1998). Ratio of Motor Nerve Conduction Velocity in Diabetic Neuropathy. *Diabetic Care* 4, pp. 615-618.

Oldfield, R. (1971). The assessment and analysis of handedness: The Edinburgh Inventory. *Neuropsychologia* 9, pp. 97-113

Olex, D. (2004). The H – reflex as an useful tool in laterality evaluation – a preliminary case study, In: . *Current research in motor control II.* Z. Waśkiewicz, G. Juras, J. Raczek. pp. 159 –162, University School of Physical Education

Olex-Zarychta, D., 2010. Neural control of the soleus H-reflex correlates to the laterality pattern in limbs. Neural Regeneration Research, 5, pp. 290-295

Olex-Zarychta, D., Koprowski, R., Sobota, G. & Wróbel, Z. (2009). Asymmetry of magnetic motor evoked potentials recorded in calf muscles of dominant and non- dominant lower extremity. *Neuroscience Letters* 465, pp. 74-78

Olex-Zarychta, D., Sobota, G., Kułdosz, J., Błaszczyk, J. (2008). Parameters of soleus H-reflex and functional laterality of lower extremities in healthy adults. In: *Current research in motor control III.* G. Juras, K. Slomka. pp. 137-146, Katowice: Academy of Physical Education in Katowice,

Olex-Zarychta, D. & Raczek, J. (2008). The relationship of movement time to hand -foot laterality patterns. *Laterality* 13 (5), pp. 439-455

Olmo, M.F., Reimunde, P., Viana, O., Acero, R.M., & Cudeiro, J. (2006). Chronic neural adaptation induced by long term resistance training in humans. *European Journal of Physiology* 96, pp. 722-728

Palmieri, R., Ingersoll, C. & Hoffmann, M. (2004). The Hoffmann reflex: methodological considerations and applications for use in sports medicine and athletic training research. *Journal of Athletic Training* 3, pp. 268-277

Pearson, K.& Gordon, J. (2000). *Spinal reflexes.* In: Kandel ER, Schwartz JH, Jessell TM. Principles of Neural Science. 9, pp.713-736. New York: McGraw-Hill

Peters, M. (1991). Laterality and motor control. *CIBA Foundation Symposium.* pp. 300-311

Rothwell, J. (1996). *Control of human voluntary movement, 2 nd edt.* London: Chapman &Hall

Roy, E.A. (1983). Manual performance asymmetries and motor control processes: subject-generated changes in response parameters. *Human Movement Science* 2, pp. 271–277

Sainburg, R.L. (2002). Evidence for a dynamic-dominance hypothesis of handedness. *Experimental Brain Research* 142, pp. 241–258

Sainburg, R.L. (2005). Handedness: differential specializations for control of trajectory and position. *Exercericise and Sport Science Review* 33, 206–213

Sarlegna, F.R., & Sainburg, R.L. (2007). The effect of target modality on visual and proprioceptive contributions to the control of movement distance. *Experimental Brain Research* 176, pp. 267-280

Schaal, S., Sternad, D., Osu, R.& Kawato, M. (2004). Rhythmic arm movement is not discrete. *Nature Neuroscience* 7 (10), pp. 1137-1144

Simonetta-Moreau, M., Marque, P., Marchand-Pauvert, V. & Pierrot-Deseilligny, E. (1999). The pattern of human lower limb motoneurones by probable group II muscle afferents. *Journal of Physiology* 517, pp. 287-300

Shabbott, B. & Sainburg, R. (2008). Differentiating between two models of motor lateralization. *Journal of Neurophysiology* 100(2), pp. 565- 575

Schabowsky, C.N., Hidler, J.M. & Lum, P.S. (2007). Greater reliance on impedance control in the nondominant arm compared with the dominant arm when adapting to a novel dynamic environment. *Experimental Brain Research* 182, pp. 567–577

Shewmann, T. (2007). *Measurement and analysis of EMG signals in clinical practice. Protocols and biofeedback in training with EMG.* WSPiA, Poznań

Sigh, P.I. & Maini, B.K. (1980). The influence of muscle use on conduction velocity of motor nerve fibers. *Indian Journal of Physiology & Pharmacology* 24(1), pp. 65-67

Springer S., Deutsch G (2004). *Left Brain, Right Brain. Perspectives from cognitive neuroscience,* 5 edn, Prószynski I S-ka SA, Warsaw

Steinmetz, H. (1996). Structure, functional and cerebral asymmetry: in vivo morphometry of the planum temporale. *Neuroscience and Biobehavioural Review* 20(4), pp. 587-591

Strauss, E. & Wada, J. (1983). Lateral preferences and cerebral speech dominance. *Cortex* 19, pp. 165-177

Tan, U. (1993). Sensory nerve conduction velocities are higher on the left than the right hand and motor conduction is faster on the right hand than left in right-handed normal subjects. *International Journal of Neuroscience* 73 (1-2), pp. 85-91

Tan, U. (1989). The H-reflex recovery curve from the wrist flexors: lateralization of motoneuronal excitability in relation to handedness in normal subjects. *International Journal of Neuroscience* 48 (3-4), pp. 271-284

Tanaka, S., Hanakawa, T., Honda, M. & Watanabe, K. (2009). Enhancement of pinch force in the lower leg by anodal transcranial direct current stimulation. *Experimental Brain Research,* 196, pp. 459- 465

Taniguchi, Y. (1999). Right hemispheric contribution to motor programing of simultaneous bilateral response. *Perceptual and Motor Skills* 88, pp. 1283-1290

Todor, J.I & Cisneros, J. (1985). Accommodation to increased accuracy demands by the right and left hands. *Journal of Motor Behaviour* 17, pp. 355–372

Toga, A. W. & Thompson, P.M. (2003). Mapping Brain Asymmetry. *Nature Reviews Neuroscience* 4, pp. 37-48

Tommasi, L. (2009). Mechanisms and functions of brain and behavioural asymmetries. *Philosophical Transactions of the Royal. Society B* 364, pp. 855-859

Tucker, K., Tuncer, M. & Türker, K. (2005). A review of the H-reflex and M-wave in the human triceps surae. *Human Movement Science* 24, pp. 667-688

Tucker, D.M. & Williamson, P.A. (1984). Asymmetric neural control systems in human self-regulation. *Psychological Review.* 91, pp. 185-215

Wang, J. & Sainburg, R. (2007). The dominant and non dominant arms are specialized for stabilizing different features of task performance. *Experimntal Brain Research* 178, pp. 565-570

Waxman, S. (2004). Determinants of conduction velocity in myelinated nerve fibers. *Muscle & Nerve* 3(2), pp.141-150

Wolpaw, J.R. & Chen, X.Y. (2006). The cerebellum in maintenance of a motor skill: a hierarchy of brain and spinal cord plasticity underlies H-reflex conditioning. *Learning & Memory* 13, pp. 208-215

Zehr, E.P. (2006). Training-induced adaptive plasticity in human somatosensory reflex pathways. *Journal of Applied Physiology* 101, pp. 1783- 1794

Zehr, P., Balter, J., Ferris, D., Hundza, S., Loadman, P. & Stoloff, R. (2007). Neural regulation of rhythmic arm and leg movement is conserved across human locomotor tasks. *Journal of Physiology* 1, pp. 209-227

Zehr, P., Carroll, T., Chua, R., Collins, D., Frigon, A., Haridas, C., Hundza, S., & Thompson, A. (2004). Possible contributions of CPG activity to the control of rhythmic human arm movements. *Canadian Journal of Physiology & Pharmacology* 82, pp. 556-568

Zieliński, K. (2006). Jerzy Konorski on brain associations. *Acta Neurobiologiae Experimentalis* 66(1), pp. 75-80

6

Underlying Causes of Paresthesia

Mahdi Sharif-Alhoseini[1], Vafa Rahimi-Movaghar[1,2] and Alexander R. Vaccaro[3]

[1]Sina Trauma and Surgery Research Center, Tehran University of Medical Sciences, Tehran,
[2]Research Centre for Neural Repair, University of Tehran, Tehran,
[3]Department of Orthopaedic Surgery, Thomas Jefferson University and Rothman Institute, Philadelphia, PA,
[1,2]Iran
[3]USA

1. Introduction

Sensations from various parts of the body are taken by the peripheral sensory nerves to the spinal cord. From spinal cord, the signals reach the brain with the help of the trigeminal nerve and brain stem. Hence, any problem in this pathway may result in paresthesia. Paresthesia is an abnormal condition which causes an individual to feel a sensation of burning, numbness, tingling, itching or prickling. It frequently happens in the extremities, but it can occur in other parts of the body as well.

The purpose of this chapter is to review the causes of paresthesia from studies indexed in PubMed. We describe the underlying conditions that may cause paresthesia based on two subdivisions: Transient and Chronic Paresthesias.

2. Causes of transient paresthesia

This paresthesia subtype involves temporary numbness or tingling that disappears quickly as can occur from sitting with your legs crossed for a long time or sleeping on your arm in a bent position. This is a very common type of paresthesia.

- Obdormition: Obdormition is a numbness caused by prolonged pressure on a nerve, such as when a leg falls asleep if the legs are crossed for a prolonged period. It disappears gradually as the pressure is relieved (1).
- Whiplash: Paresthesias in the upper extremity may occur after whiplash injury (2), a type of cervical soft tissue injury (3). Pujol et al showed that 13% of patients with whiplash had associated paresthesias (4). Recovery usually arises within 6 months after injury (5).
- Hyperventilation syndrome: Paresthesia constitutes 35% of presenting complaints in patients with hyperventilation syndrome (6) and may begin after as little as three-minute of hyperventilation (7). After increasing the depth or frequency of respiration,

the alkaline shift produced selectively increases Na^+ conductance and ectopic discharges in normal cutaneous afferent nerves can be induced (8). Other electrolytes, i.e. magnesium, potassium, chloride, phosphate and bicarbonate, also demonstrated significant changes in concentration (7).

- Panic attack: Paresthesiae of the mouth, hands and feet are common, transient symptoms of the related conditions of hyperventilation syndrome and panic attacks. Ietsugu et al demonstrated that paresthesia can be used as a reliable indicator of severe panic attacks (9).
- Transient ischemic attack (TIA): TIA may be manifested by paresthesias. Several reasons may cause TIA such as thrombosis, embolus, intravascular debris and blood vessels disruption. Perez et al. reported the initial manifestation of cardiac myxoma can be paresthesias caused by TIA (10). Post-ischemic paresthesia occurs when hyper polarization by the Na^+/K^+ pump is transiently halted by elevated extracellular K^+. The electrochemical gradient for K^+ is reversed and inward transport of K^+ triggers regenerative depolarization (8).
- Seizures: Paresthesia may happen during and after a partial seizure (11). Treatment of seizures with vagus nerve stimulation can also trigger paresthesias and is considered an adverse event associated with this treatment modality (12).
- Dehydration: At around 5% to 6% cumulative water loss, paresthesia may occur.
- Insufficient blood supply: Circulatory disorders could lead to transient or chronic paresthesia.

Acute arterial occlusion by an embolism or in situ thrombosis is a dramatic event which produces severe ischemia of distal tissue. The warning signs are the 5 Ps: pallor, pain, pulselessness, paralysis and paresthesia. In such cases, emergent restoration of blood flow by surgery may be vital to prevent limb loss (13). Aneurysms and dilated forms of atherosclerosis can be both the cause of in situ thrombosis as well as the source of an embolism (14).

In Buerger's disease (thromboangiitis obliterans), an occlusive intraluminal thrombus with a predominantly acute inflammatory infiltrate causes ischemic ulcers, claudication, paresthesia and pain at rest (15, 16).

Raynaud's syndrome describes a condition characterized by the sensation of coldness, burning pain or numbness in the fingers or toes. This syndrome occurs when the blood vessels in the fingers or toes spasm, restricting the flow of blood. Some causative factors can activate Raynaud's syndrome including contact to cold and emotional stress (17, 18).

- Apheresis: Because of improvements in technique and instrumentation used for apheresis, symptoms of mild ionized hypocalcemia, such as paresthesias or lightheadedness, are increasingly easily manageable and quickly reversible with flow-rate adjustments. Puig et al. reported a 2.27 percent incidence of paresthesia in therapeutic apheresis (19).
- Beta-alanine ingestion: Beta-alanine supplementation is used as a nutritional strategy to improve high-intensity anaerobic performance (20). Paresthesia may be observed if a single dose higher than 800 mg is ingested but is transient and abates as plasma concentration declines. This side effect can be prevented by using controlled release capsules and smaller dosing strategies (21).

3. Causes of chronic paresthesia

Chronic paresthesia or intermittent paresthesia over a long period of time is generally a sign of neurological disease or traumatic nerve damage. Paresthesia usually arises from nerve damage due to infection, inflammation, trauma, or other abnormal process. Paresthesia is rarely due to life-threatening disorders, but it can occur as a result of stroke and tumors. Whereas paresthesia is a loss of sensation, paralysis usually involves both a loss of movement and sensation.

- Nervous System Disorders

Paresthesias are common manifestations of central and peripheral pathological processes and are due to ectopic impulse activity in cutaneous afferents or their central projections (8).

- Central nervous system etiologies
  In the central nervous system, the most common etiologies of paresthesia include ischemia, compressive phenomena, infection, inflammation, and degenerative conditions (22).
  - Stroke: Paresthesia and sensory deficits are considered as signs of stroke (23). In unusual cases, mandibular or ear paresthesia may be the only presenting symptom of a cerebrovascular accident (24). A persistent unpleasant numbness after a cerebrovascular accident can result from central poststroke paresthesia (25).
  - Paresthesia may be caused by selective lacunar infarcts in the diencephalic and mesencephalic regions or in the diaschisis in the parietal cortex. Chang and Huang reported a patient who presented with unilateral paresthesia after acute isolated infarct of the splenium (26). Kim reported that paresthesia or pain occurred between 0 to 24 months after lenticulocapsular hemorrhage, more prominently in the leg than other body parts (27). In another case report, a thalamic lacunar infarct led to sudden isolated left-sided paresthesia involving the face, upper and lower limbs (28). Cheiro-oral syndrome is characterized by paresthesia and sensory impairment confined to the perioral region and ipsilateral fingers or hand, and arises from small stroke-related lesions to various sites between the medulla and cortex (29).
  - Intra-cerebral hemorrhage: Paresthesia is a symptom of acute intra-cerebral hematoma (30). Epidural or subdural hematoma or subarachnoid hemorrhage should be considered as part of the differential diagnosis for acute paresthesia and extremity weakness (31-33). Kishida et al. reported that a small hematoma localized in the ventroposterior lateral nucleus caused paresthesia limited to the forearm and the palm (34).
  - Brain tumor: A sudden numbness especially when accompanied by headache, nausea or vomiting, double vision, or weakness could suggest a possible brain tumor or metastasis (35). Cavernous angioma which typically presents with neurological deficits, low back pain and sciatica or as a subarachnoid hemorrhage could be a cause of paresthesia (36). A small round tumor of the somatosensory cortex may present with radicular hand pain and paresthesia (37). Trigeminal sensory neuropathy presents with anesthesia and paresthesia of the orofacial region may herald underlying malignancy (38). Syringomyelia, which is generally related to congenital malformations and tumors, may lead to paresthesia (39).

- Head trauma: Brain injury patients report high rates of complaints generally recognized as being associated with neuropsychological impairment such as paresthesia (40). Trigeminal trophic syndrome is an unusual complication after peripheral or central damage to the trigeminal nerve, characterized by anesthesia, paresthesias, and ala nasi ulceration. It can be preceded by head trauma, iatrogenic injury or other causes (41, 42).
- Encephalitis and meningitis: Brain inflammations may lead to paresthesia (43). Eosinophilic meningitis is typically induced by the nematode Angiostrongylus cantonensis and presents with headache, vomiting and fever, and may also induce paresthesia and neck stiffness (44).
- Abscess: A primary brain abscess may begin with neurologic deficit such as paresthesia (45, 46).
- Lumbar spinal stenosis: 70% of patients experience paresthesia which is exacerbated by extension, and improves with spinal flexion (47, 48).
- Systemic lupus erythematosus: Systemic vasculitis may present with multiple neurologic and psychiatric symptoms due to involvement of the central and peripheral nervous systems. Painful paresthesias and weakness of the limbs have been reported in cases of systemic lupus erythematosus (49, 50).
- Multiple sclerosis: One of the most common presenting symptoms in Multiple Sclerosis is paresthesia (51, 52). About 40% of the patients reported that such symptoms had an important adverse influence on daily activities. Painful paresthesia leads to avoidance of any triggering activities (53).
- Transverse myelitis: Sensory impairment and paresthesia in the extremities are two common presentations of acute transverse myelitis (54-57). That is a relatively uncommon neurological disease in which affected patients exhibit acute dehabilitating symptoms associated with the loss of spinal cord segment function.
- Spinal puncture: Paresthesia rarely occurs during spinal puncture or injection of local anesthetic for spinal anesthesia (58). A paresthesia may result from needle-to-nerve contact with a spinal nerve in the epidural space, or, with far lateral needle placement, such as during placement of a spinal needle into the intervertebral foramen (59). It seems that lateral decubitus position results in a higher incidence of paresthesiae than the sitting position (60).
- Vitamin B_{12} deficiency: Neurological symptoms such as paresthesia are frequent in vitamin B_{12} deficiency (61, 62). However therapeutic response to vitamin B_{12} with resolution of associated symptoms is dramatic (63).

- Peripheral nervous system etiologies (with or without pain)

The most common source of paresthesia is peripheral neuropathy.

Cutaneous afferents nerves are more volatile than motor axons, due to differences in their biophysical properties. These differences maybe include more persistent Na^+ conductance and inward rectification on cutaneous afferents, properties which probably give greater protection from impulse-dependent conduction failure but produce a greater tendency for ectopic activity (8).

- Entrapment neuropathies

Numbness and paresthesia are two more common complaints in patients with peripheral neuropathies (64).

  - Carpal tunnel syndrome: Carpal tunnel syndrome is the most common entrapment neuropathy caused by compression of the median nerve within the carpal tunnel. It is characterized by pain and paresthesia, with a usual night exacerbation and aggravation by activity along the distribution of the median nerve (65-67).
  - Lateral femoral cutaneous syndrome: Meralgia paresthetica is a rarely encountered sensory mononeuropathy characterized by paresthesia, pain or sensory impairment along the distribution of the lateral femoral cutaneous nerve (LFCN) caused by entrapment or compression of the nerve as it crosses the anterior superior iliac spine and runs beneath the inguinal ligament. Ultrasound-guided blockade of the LFCN is a safe and success technique to treat this condition (68, 69).
  - Isolated femoral neuropathy: This neuropathy occurs due to direct compression of the femoral nerve, indirect compression by the psoas muscle during pelvic surgery, direct ischemia of the nerve by clamping of the iliac artery during the vascular anastomosis or vessel dissection, or by postoperative hematoma in the retroperitoneum or psoas muscle. Isolated femoral neuropathy causes numbness and paresthesia located in the anteromedial part of the thigh (70).
  - Tarsal tunnel syndrome: Paresthesia in the foot is the most frequent symptom of tarsal tunnel syndrome and may have an arterial etiology (71). Kim and Childers suggested ultrasound-guided injection of 0.5% lidocaine to temporarily resolve the paresthesia as a diagnostic modality (72).
- Sciatica: Sciatica is commonly due to a prolapsed intervertebral disc, although spinal canal stenosis, spondylolisthesis, piriformis syndrome, spinal tumours and other causes must be considered. Leg pain, paresthesia and weakness are the most bothersome symptoms in sciatica (73-75).
- Disc herniation: Radicular compression by a disc herniation may lead to the radiating paresthesia into the extremities (76, 77)
- Cervical spondylosis: Hand paresthesia is a frequent and early symptom found in patients either with cervical spondylosis or carpal tunnel syndrome (78). In cervical spondylosis, paresthesia is not commonly nocturnal, aggravated by hand activity, or associated with hand pain, in contrast to carpal tunnel syndrome (67).
- Pressure palsy: Paresthesia may be a presenting complaint in pressure palsy (79). Hereditary neuropathy with liability to pressure palsies (HNPP) is an autosomal-dominant inherited disease clinically characterized by painless and episodic or recurrent neurological symptoms such as peripheral palsy or paresthesia, often preceded by minor trauma or toxic damage (80, 81). However, the presence of mild symptoms and the marked phenotypic variability of the disease result in underdiagnosis of HNPP (82).
- Charcot-Marie-Tooth disease: Charcot-Marie-Tooth hereditary neuropathy refers to a group of disorders characterized by a chronic motor and sensory polyneuropathy (83). The affected individual typically has distal muscle weakness and atrophy often associated with mild to moderate sensory loss, depressed tendon reflexes, high-arched feet, severe cramps and painful paresthesia (83, 84)

    - Amyloid neuropathy: In 1975, Kyle and Bayrd investigated 236 cases of amyloidosis and reported that paresthesia was one of the most common presenting symptoms besides fatigue, light-headedness and weight loss (85). Paresthesia may have a glove and stocking or even thoraco-abdominal distribtuion (86).
    - Repetitive motion or prolonged vibration: Nerve compression in repetitive motion disorders is being recognized with increasing frequency. The pathophysiology of chronic nerve compression spans a broad spectrum beginning with subperineurial edema and progressing to axonal degeneration. The changes seen depend on the amount and duration of the compressive forces and lead to pain, tingling, numbness and paresthesia (87).
    - Neuralgia: Neuralgia is a painful sensation in one or multiple nerve distribution which can be mild or severe, and acute or chronic. Many patients with neuropathic pain exhibit persistent or paroxysmal pain and paresthesias that are independent of any stimulus (88).
    - Removal of impacted mandibular third molars (M3s): Extraction of impacted M3s may cause temporary or permanent neurosensorial disturbances of the inferior alveolar and lingual nerves (89, 90).
- Circulatory disorders (As mentioned before, insufficient blood supply could lead to transient or chronic paresthesia).
- Thoracic outlet syndrome (TOS)
  - Arterial TOS. The symptoms of Arterial TOS include digital ischemia, claudication, pallor, coldness, paresthesia and pain in the hand but seldom in the shoulder or neck. These symptoms are the result of arterial emboli arising either from mural thrombus in a subclavian artery aneurysm or from a thrombus forming just distal to a focus of subclavian artery stenosis.
  - Venous TOS. Paresthesia in the fingers and hands is common in venous TOS and may be secondary to swelling in the hand rather than to nerve compression in the thoracic outlet area.
  - Neurogenic TOS. Pain, paresthesia, and weakness in the hand, arm, and shoulder, plus neck pain and occipital headaches are the classical symptoms of Neurogenic TOS. Raynaud's phenomenon, hand coldness and color changes is also frequently seen in NTOS. It is the latter symptoms that can lead to an erroneous diagnosis of Arterial TOS (91).
- Metabolic disorders
  - Diabetes: The most common causes of paresthesia in the United States are diabetes and alcoholism (22). Sensory nerve dysfunction is a progressive form of diabetic neuropathy, and is often accompanied by other microvascular complications. This complication is more common in middle aged and elderly men with type 2 diabetes mellitus (92).
  - Alcoholism: The most common complication of chronic alcohol intake is a toxic polyneuropathy. Nutritional deficiency as well as the direct neurotoxic effects of ethanol or its metabolites can cause alcoholic neuropathy (93). This neuropathy is manifested by distal sensory disturbances with pain and paresthesia in a glove and stocking pattern (94).
  - Hypoglycemia: Specific symptoms and signs may vary by age, the severity of the hypoglycemia and the speed of the decline in blood sugar. Paresthesia may be a

neuroglycopenic or adrenergic manifestations of hypoglycemia. Recurrent hypoglycemia which is commonly seen in patients with an insulinoma causes periodic weakness, vertigo and perioral paresthesia (95).

- Hypothyroidism: Paresthesia is a more frequent clinical manifestation observed in hypothyroidism (96, 97). About 40% of hypothyroid patients have predominantly sensory signs of a sensorimotor axonal neuropathy early in the course of thyroid disease. It appears that the axonal myelin sheath begins to degenerate without sufficient thyroid hormone, and regeneration of damaged nerves also slows (98).
- Hypoparathyroidism: Hypoparathyroidism is the most common cause of hypocalcemia. Acute hypocalcemia causes increased neuromuscular irritability which in milder forms lead to paresthesia and numbness of acral and perioral areas (99, 100).
- Hyperaldosteronism: Most clinical effects of hyperaldoste-ronism result from hypokalemia, which increases neuromuscular irritability and produces weakness, paralysis, and paresthesia (101).
- Menopause: One of the most common reported somatic symptoms is paresthesia in the extremities (102). Decreasing estrogen production causes decreased structural effectiveness of collagen and thinning of the skin. This leads to reduced blow flow to the superficial nerves and symptoms of numbness and tingling (103).
- Abnormal blood levels of calcium, potassium or sodium *(See Hyperventilation syndrome in Causes of transient paresthesia)*
- Uremia: Polyneuropathy is one of the most frequent manifestations in chronic uremia. Hemodialyzed uremic patients have been found to have vitamin B_6 deficiency which may lead to paresthesia (104). Uremia can also cause restless legs syndrome which is clinically defined as an urge to move the legs with or without associated paresthesia (105).
- Porphyria: The most common symptoms of porphyria are abdominal pain, peripheral polyneuropathy, flaccid paresis, with or without autonomic involvement (106). Nerve biopsy shows segmental demyelination and axonal degeneration and also many small vacuolations are seen in the cell body of affected nerves (107).
- Amyloidosis (*See Amyloid neuropathy in Peripheral nervous system etiologies)*

- Infections and post-infection syndromes
  - Herpes simplex virus: Herpetic infection causes paresthesia. Immunohistochemical studies suggest that sensory ganglion infection occurs via centripetal axonal migration of the virus (108). Topical caffeine can inhibit this paresthesia through direct action on sensory neurons (109).
  - Herpes zoster virus: Primary infection by varicella-zoster virus (VZV) may be associated with several neurologic complications such as paresthesia (110, 111). VZV remains dormant in dorsal root and cranial nerve ganglia and can be reactivated as a consequence of declining VZV-specific cellular immunity leading to herpes zoster (shingles) (112). Following reactivation, centrifugal migration of herpes zoster virus occurs along sensory nerves to produce a characteristic painful cutaneous or mucocutaneous vesicular eruption that is generally limited to the affected dermatome (113). The commonest prodromes are pain, itching and paresthesia (114-116)

- Canker sores: Canker sores or apthous ulcers are painful and round white sores with a red border that occur inside the mouth. There is a tingling or burning sensation prior to the appearance of the sores. They are associated with various nutritional and immunological deficiencies. However, they are more common in individuals with acute HIV infection (117, 118).
- Lyme disease: Lyme disease, caused by the tick-borne spirochete Borrelia burgdorferi, is associated with a wide variety of neurologic manifestations. Neuropathic symptoms such as symmetric, distal and nonpainful paresthesia, and asymmetric radicular pain begin 8 months after erythema migrans occurs and are present for up to 12 months (119, 120)
- Human Immunodeficiency Virus type-1 (HIV-1): Peripheral neuropathies commonly complicate all stages of the HIV-1 disease. Whereas symptomatic neuropathies occur in approximately 10% to 15% of HIV-1-infected patients overall, pathologic evidence of peripheral nerve involvement is present in virtually all end-stage AIDS patients. The dominant clinical features in distal sensory polyneuropathy which is the most common among the HIV-1-associated neuropathies include distal pain, paresthesia and numbness in a typical length-dependent fashion with a proximal to distal gradient (121, 122).
- Leprosy: Leprosy is a slowly progressive, chronic infectious disease caused by the bacillus Mycobacterium leprae. The skin and peripheral nerves are the most commonly affected organs (123). Predominant presenting symptoms are paresthesia, pain and sensory/motor deficit (124).
- Syphilis: Neurosyphilis may cause paresthesia (125, 126). Paresthesia can be due to spinal myelitis caused by neurosyphilis (127).
- Guillain-Barré syndrome (GBS): GBS is an acute, symmetrical polyneuropathy with distinctive features. The early clinical course involves painful paresthesia that is usually followed by proximal motor weakness (128). Some infectious pathogens may play a role in the pathogenesis of GBS (129).
- Rabies: Rabies, which is an acute, progressive, fatal zoonotic infectious disease, is almost always caused by the bite of rabid animals (130, 131). The rabies virus travels to the brain by following the peripheral nerves. Once the rabies virus reaches the central nervous system and symptoms begin to show, the infection is effectively untreatable and usually fatal within days. Early-stage symptoms of rabies are malaise, headache and fever, progressing to acute pain, paresthesia, violent movements and hydrophobia (132).

- Autoimmune diseases
  - Rheumatoid arthritis: Dry mouth, pruritus and paresthesia are frequent complaints in patients with rheumatoid arthritis (133). Rheumatoid cervical myelopathy causes paresthesia in the arms and neck pain (134).
  - Systemic lupus erythematosus *(See Systemic lupus erythematosus in Central nervous system etiologies)*
  - Sjogren's syndrome: Peripheral neuropathy occurs in Sjogren's syndrome. The history often reveals complaints of burning, tingling paresthesias in a symmetrical stocking or glove distribution or in the face (Trigeminal Nerve) area (135-137).
  - Pernicious anemia *(See Vitamin B_{12} deficiency in Central nervous system etiologies)*
  - Diabetes *(See Diabetes in Methabolic disorders)*

- Arthritis: The involvement of the cervical spine is the most serious skeletal manifestation of rheumatoid arthritis. In patients with basilar impression and/or rheumatoid cervical myelopathy, paresthesia in the upper limbs was significantly more common (134, 138). Paresthesia can occur in psoriatic arthritis (139).
- Fibromyalgia: Fibromyalgia is a frequent disorder of the middle aged, particularly in women characterized by chronic, diffuse musculoskeletal pain and by a low pain threshold at specific anatomical points (tender points) (140). Cacace et al. found that paresthesia had the highest frequency among associated clinical distress in fibromyalgia (141).
- Nutrient deficiency
- Vitamin B_1: Thiamine (vitamin B_1) deficiency leads to Beri-Beri which takes two forms. Dry beri-beri has symptoms of peripheral neuropathy with ataxia, weakness, paresthesia, and patchy sensory loss with areflexia (142).
- Vitamin B_5: It seems that pantothenic acid (vitamin B_5) can cause sensory polyneuropathy (143).
- Vitamin B_6: The symptoms related to pyridoxine (vitamin B_6) deficiency are peripheral neuropathies, such as paresthesia and burning dysesthesias (104).
- Vitamin B_{12} (See Vitamin B_{12} deficiency in Central nervous system etiologies)
- Malignancies: Local paresthesia can be caused by a malignancy which puts pressure on adjacent nerves. For example a reported osteosarcoma in the left segment of the maxilla led to swelling and paresthesia in the left cheek (144), and periorbital paresthesia is usually a sign of malignancy (145). Multiple myeloma with extraosseous lesions may result in paresthesia of soft tissue (146). On the other hand the association between polyneuropathy and multiple myeloma as the result of various clinical variants should be considered (147). POEMS syndrome which is identified as Polyneuropathy, Organomegaly, Endocrinopathy, Monoclonal Gammopathy and Skin changes, presents with abdominal distension, progressive paresthesia and motor weakness of both lower extremities (148).
- Skin disorders
- Burns: Studies of patients recovering from significant burns show that abnormal sensations such as paresthesia are frequently reported as long as several years after the injury (149, 150). Furthermore long-term paresthesia is a complication reported after electrical burns (151, 152).
- Frostbite: Frostbite injuries occur mainly in the toes, fingers, ears, nose and cheek. Typically an initial vasoconstriction in the skin will protect against drop in core temperature. Ice crystal development occurs when tissue temperature drops to -2° C, leading to increased osmolality of the extracellular fluid and intracellular dehydration. White-cyanotic discoloration, pain and paresthesia followed by hypoesthesia are the symptoms of frostbite injury (153).
- Ito syndrome: Hypomelanosis of Ito is a rare neurocutaneous disorder. It is characterized by depigmented skin areas often associated with ocular, musculoskeletal and neurological abnormalities (154).
- Pink disease: Acrodynia (pink disease) occurs in children exposed to mercury for prolonged periods (155). Affected patients are initially listless, anorexic, and

irritable. Their blood pressure and heart rate increase. Significant pain occurs in the hands and feet preventing sleep. Finally the hands and feet will swell and become paresthetic, becoming a dusky pink color along with a similar process which occurs in the nose (156).

- Acroparesthesia: Postmenopausal women may experience acroparesthesia. Hormone therapy can increase forearm/hand blood flow, and help ameliorate these symptoms (157).
  - Migraine: The somatosensory aura of a migraine may consist of digitolingual or cheiro-oral paresthesias. The paresthesia may migrate up the arm and then extend to involve the face, lips and tongue (158).
  - Psychological disorders: Anxiety, panic attack and psychiatric diseases may cause hyperventilation which can lead to paresthesia (6). Paresthesia also can be a manifestation of depression (159).
  - Medications: Paresthesia can be a side effect of some medications such as anti-convulsant drugs, topiramate, amiodarone, digoxin, dimercaprol, colistimethate, mefloquine, metronidazole, HIV medications, riluzole, tetrodotoxin, thallium, vincristine, diphenoxylate, overdose of lidocain or vitamin B_6 (1). Sertraline can induce facial paresthesia (160). SSRI withdrawal may cause paresthesia. The neurotoxicity of immuno-suppressive agents (e.g. calcineurin-inhibitors) may cause mild symptoms, such as tremors and paresthesia (161). Motexafin lutetium which is used in the treatment of coronary atherosclerosis or vulnerable plaque can cause the paresthesia (23).
  - Toxins
- Alcohol (See Alcoholism in Metabolic disorders)
- Tobacco: Smoking is a strong risk factor for arteriosclerosis and Buerger's disease which can cause sensitive axonal polyneuropathy (15, 162).
- Drug abuse: Intravenous administrating of strong pharmaceutical drugs acting on the central nervous system, mainly opioids especially in non-medical use (drug abuse) can lead to neurological manifestations such as paresthesia (1).
- Heavy metals
  - Mercury: toxicity from organic mercurials includes neurologic decompensation with mental deterioration, ataxia, spasms, paresthesia, deafness, and eventually coma (156).
  - Arsenic: Neurological and neurophysiological studies indicate that the functions of the central and peripheral nervous system may be impaired under conditions of exposure to arsenic (163).
  - Lead: The prominent findings among the lead-exposed workers are fatigue, abdominal discomfort, backache, myalgia and paresthesia (164).
- Nitrous oxide: Exposure to nitrous oxide may damage the nervous system which can lead to ascending paresthesia of the limbs, severe ataxia of gait, tactile sensory loss on the limbs and trunk, and absent tendon reflexes (165, 166).
- Carbon monoxide: Paresthesia, emesis, diarrhea, unilateral headache, palpitation or death are non-specific but common symptoms of carbon monoxide poisoning (167).
- Snake bites: Some venom contains toxins which attack the nervous system, causing neurotoxicity. The victim may present with strange disturbances to their vision, paresthesia, difficulty speaking and respiratory paralysis (168).

- Ciguatera: Ciguatera is the most frequently observed form of tropical fish poisoning. It blocks the sodium channel leading to slowed nerve conduction and causes the peripheral and central nervous system symptoms such as facial paresthesia, myalgia, cramps and weakness. Ciguatera poisoning leads to the gastrointestinal and cardiovascular disturbances too (169, 170).
  - Radiation exposure: Chronic progressive radiation myelopathy develops with a latency of several months to years after spinal cord irradiation. The symptoms are paresthesia, paresis or paralysis, leading to severe physical disability (171).
  - Chemotherapy: Intrathecal injections of cytarabine and methotrexate can lead to paresthesias and weakness causing patient to be wheelchair bound (172).
  - Hereditary diseases
- Fabry disease: Fabry syndrome is a genetic disease related to changes on the X chromosome. It is caused by deficient activity of alpha-galactosidase A and is characterized by intralysosomal storage of glycosphingolipids. The main clinical features are paresthesia, hypohidrosis, angiokeratoma, renal insufficiency, and cardiovascular or cerebral complications (173, 174).
- Refsum syndrome: Refsum's disease is an autosomal recessive disorder with clinical features that include retinitis pigmentosa, blindness, anosmia, deafness, sensory neuropathy, ataxia and accumulation of phytanic acid in plasma- and lipid-containing tissues (175).
- Charcot-Marie-Tooth disease *(See Charcot-Marie-Tooth disease in Peripheral nervous system etiologies)*
- Porphyria *(See Porphyria in Metabolic disorders)*
- Ataxia-teleangiectasia: Ataxia-telangiectasia is a progressive neurodegenerative disorder, with onset in early childhood. It is an autosomal recessive disorder that includes progressive cerebellar ataxia, dysarthric speech, oculomotor apraxia, choreoathetosis and, later, oculocutaneous telangiectasia (176, 177).
  - Immune deficiency: The immune response dysfunction induced by the human immunodeficiency virus infection sometimes causes inflammatory lesions of the central and peripheral nervous system leading to neurological symptoms such as paresthesia (178).

4. References

[1] Modric J. Causes of Tingling and Numbness - Paresthesia. 2011; http://www.healthhype.com [cited 2011 June 8]

[2] Hadziahmetovic Z, Vavra-Hadziahmetovic N. Whiplash neck injury. Med Arh. 2008;62(4):215-7. [Bosnian]

[3] Ferrari R, Russell AS, Carroll LJ, Cassidy JD. A re-examination of the whiplash associated disorders (WAD) as a systemic illness. Ann Rheum Dis. 2005 ;64(9):1337-42.

[4] Pujol A, Puig L, Mansilla J, Idiaquez I. Relevant factors in medico-legal prognosis of whiplash injury. Med Clin (Barc). 2003;121(6):209-15.[Spanish]

[5] Karnezis I, Drosos G, Kazakos K. Factors affecting the timing of recovery from whiplash neck injuries: study of a cohort of 134 patients pursuing litigation. Archives of Orthopaedic and Trauma Surgery. 2007;127(8):633-6.

[6] Saisch SG, Wessely S, Gardner WN. Patients with acute hyperventilation presenting to an inner-city emergency department. Chest. 1996;110(4):952-7.

[7] Stadler G, Steurer J, Dur P, Binswanger U, Vetter W. Electrolyte changes during and after voluntary hyperventilation. Praxis (Bern 1994). 1995;84(12):328-34. [German]
[8] Mogyoros I, Bostock H, Burke D. Mechanisms of paresthesias arising from healthy axons. Muscle & Nerve. 2000;23(3):310-20.
[9] Ietsugu T, Sukigara M, Furukawa TA. Evaluation of diagnostic criteria for panic attack using item response theory: Findings from the National Comorbidity Survey in USA. Journal of Affective Disorders. 2007;104(1-3):197-201.
[10] Perez de Colosia Rama V, Boveda Alvarez FJ, Zabala YMMS, Lucini Pelayo G. [Ischemic stroke and cardiac myxomas. Findings in cranial magnetic resonance imaging]. Neurologia. 2006;21(5):260-4.
[11] Devinsky O, Kelley K, Porter RJ, Theodore WH. Clinical and electroencephalographic features of simple partial seizures. Neurology. 1988;38(9):1347-52.
[12] Privitera MD, Welty TE, Ficker DM, Welge J. Vagus nerve stimulation for partial seizures. Cochrane Database Syst Rev. 2002(1):CD002896.
[13] Stirnemann P. Surgical therapy of acute and chronic arterial occlusions below the inguinal ligament. Praxis (Bern 1994). 2001;90(4):113-8. [German]
[14] Largiader J, Schneider E. Therapy of acute peripheral arterial occlusion. Herz. 1991;16(6):456-62.[German]
[15] Salimi J, Tavakkoli H, Salimzadeh A, Ghadimi H, Habibi G, Masoumi AA. Clinical characteristics of Buerger's disease in Iran. J Coll Physicians Surg Pak. 2008;18(8):502-5.
[16] Goiriz-Valdes R, Fernandez-Herrera J. Buerger's disease (thromboangiitis obliterans). Actas Dermosifiliogr. 2005;96(9):553-62. [Spanish]
[17] Harper F, Maricq H, Turner R, Lidman R, Leroy E. A prospective study of raynaud phenomenon and early connective tissue disease: A five-year report. The American journal of medicine. 1982;72(6):883-8.
[18] Chandler S. What Are the Causes of Numb Toes? 2011; http://www.livestrong.com/article/ [cited 2011 June 10]
[19] Puig L, Mazzara R, Torras A, Castillo R. Adverse effects secondary to the treatment with plasma exchange. Int J Artif Organs. 1985;8(3):155-8.
[20] Sale C, Saunders B, Harris RC. Effect of beta-alanine supplementation on muscle carnosine concentrations and exercise performance. Amino Acids. 2010;39(2):321-33.
[21] Artioli GG, Gualano B, Smith A, Stout J, Lancha AH, Jr. Role of beta-alanine supplementation on muscle carnosine and exercise performance. Med Sci Sports Exerc. 2010;42(6):1162-73.
[22] McKnight JT, Adcock BB. Paresthesias: a practical diagnostic approach. Am Fam Physician. 1997;56(9):2253-60.
[23] Kereiakes DJ, Szyniszewski AM, Wahr D, Herrmann HC, Simon DI, Rogers C, et al. Phase I drug and light dose-escalation trial of motexafin lutetium and far red light activation (phototherapy) in subjects with coronary artery disease undergoing percutaneous coronary intervention and stent deployment: procedural and long-term results. Circulation. 2003;108(11):1310-5.
[24] Nelson LW, Johnson WT, Blaha DA. Mandibular paresthesia secondary to cerebrovascular changes. Oral Surg Oral Med Oral Pathol. 1986;62(1):17-9.
[25] Ong CT, Sung SF, Wu CS, Lo CN. An Open-label Study of Amitriptyline in Central Poststroke Paresthesia. Acta Neurologica Taiwanica. 2003;12(4):177-80.

[26] Chang TP, Huang CF. Unilateral paresthesia after isolated infarct of the splenium: case report. Acta Neurol Taiwan. 2010;19(2):116-9.
[27] Kim JS. Central post-stroke pain or paresthesia in lenticulocapsular hemorrhages. Neurology. 2003;61(5):679-82.
[28] Rondepierre P, De Reuck J, Leclerc X, Steinling M, Godefroy O, Terrasi J, et al. Pure sensory stroke revealing a complex malformation of extra- and intracranial cerebral arteries. Clin Neurol Neurosurg. 1993;95(4):297-302.
[29] Chen WH. Cheiro-oral syndrome: a clinical analysis and review of literature. Yonsei Med J. 2009;50(6):777-83.
[30] Sengul G, Tuzun Y, Kadioglu HH, Aydin IH. Acute interhemispheric subdural hematoma due to hemodialysis: case report. Surg Neurol. 2005;64 Suppl 2:S113-4.
[31] Lo MD. Spinal cord injury from spontaneous epidural hematoma: report of 2 cases. Pediatr Emerg Care. 2010;26(6):445-7.
[32] Cho DC, Sung JK. Traumatic subacute spinal subdural hematoma successfully treated with lumbar drainage: case report. J Spinal Disord Tech. 2009;22(1):73-6.
[33] Delalande S, De Seze J, Hurtevent JP, Stojkovic T, Hurtevent JF, Vermersch P. Cortical blindness associated with Guillain-Barre syndrome: a complication of dysautonomia?. Rev Neurol (Paris). 2005;161(4):465-7. [French]
[34] Kishida Y, Maeshima S, Morita Y, Makabe T, Kunishio K, Tsubahara A. A case of recurrence of cerebral hemorrhage in a patient with adult moyamoya disease in the recovery period rehabilitation ward. No To Shinkei. 2006;58(4):319-22. [Japanese]
[35] Yang HD, Lee KH. Medullary Hemorrhage after Ischemic Wallenberg's Syndrome in a Patient with Cavernous Angioma. J Clin Neurol. 2010;6(4):221-3.
[36] Er U, Yigitkanli K, Simsek S, Adabag A, Bavbek M. Spinal intradural extramedullary cavernous angioma: case report and review of the literature. Spinal Cord. 2007;45(9):632-6.
[37] Khalatbari M, Ghalenoui H, Yahyavi ST, Borghei-Razavi H. Left somatosensory cortex tumor presented with radicular hand pain and paresthesia. Arch Iran Med. 2008;11(1):107-9.
[38] Shotts RH, Porter SR, Kumar N, Scully C. Longstanding trigeminal sensory neuropathy of nontraumatic cause. Oral Surg Oral Med Oral Pathol Oral Radiol Endod. 1999;87(5):572-6.
[39] Sahin S, Comert A, Akin O, Ayalp S, Karsidag S. Painless burn injury caused by post-traumatic syringomyelia. Ir J Med Sci. 2008;177(4):405-7.
[40] Lees-Haley PR, Brown RS. Neuropsychological complaint base rates of 170 personal injury claimants. Arch Clin Neuropsychol. 1993;8(3):203-9.
[41] Kautz O, Bruckner-Tuderman L, Muller ML, Schempp CM. Trigeminal trophic syndrome with extensive ulceration following herpes zoster. Eur J Dermatol. 2009;19(1):61-3.
[42] Monrad SU, Terrell JE, Aronoff DM. The trigeminal trophic syndrome: an unusual cause of nasal ulceration. J Am Acad Dermatol. 2004;50(6):949-52.
[43] Reynaud L, Graf M, Gentile I, Cerini R, Ciampi R, Noce S, et al. A rare case of brainstem encephalitis by Listeria monocytogenes with isolated mesencephalic localization. Case report and review. Diagn Microbiol Infect Dis. 2007;58(1):121-3.
[44] Kittimongkolma S, Intapan PM, Laemviteevanich K, Kanpittaya J, Sawanyawisuth K, Maleewong W. Eosinophilic meningitis associated with angiostrongyliasis: clinical features, laboratory investigations and specific diagnostic IgG and IgG subclass antibodies in cerebrospinal fluid. Southeast Asian J Trop Med Public Health. 2007;38(1):24-31.

[45] Malincarne L, Marroni M, Farina C, Camanni G, Valente M, Belfiori B, et al. Primary brain abscess with Nocardia farcinica in an immunocompetent patient. Clin Neurol Neurosurg. 2002;104(2):132-5.
[46] Nakaya M, Okimoto M, Abe H, Sato A, Watanabe Y, Nakajima N. A mitral valve reconstruction of infective endocarditis with brain abscess and intracranial mycotic aneurysm. Jpn J Thorac Cardiovasc Surg. 1998;46(7):647-50. [Japanese]
[47] Oniankitan O, Magnan A, Fianyo E, Mijiyawa M. Lumbar spinal stenosis in an outpatient clinic in Lome, Togo. Med Trop (Mars). 2007;67(3):263-6. [French]
[48] Nowakowski P, Delitto A, Erhard RE. Lumbar spinal stenosis. Phys Ther. 1996;76(2):187-90.
[49] Harscher S, Rummler S, Oelzner P, Mentzel HJ, Brodhun M, Witte OW, et al. [Selective immunoadsorption in neurologic complications of systemic lupus erythematosus]. Nervenarzt. 2007;78(4):441-4.
[50] Ilniczky S, Kamondi A, Aranyi Z, Varallyay G, Gaal B, Szirmai I, et al. Simultaneous central and peripheral nervous system involvement in systemic lupus erythematosus. Ideggyogy Sz. 2007;60(9-10):398-402.
[51] Ashtari F, Shaygannejad V, Farajzadegan Z, Amin A. Does early-onset multiple sclerosis differ from adult-onset form in Iranian people. J Res Med Sci. 2010 Mar;15(2):94-9.
[52] Beiske AG, Pedersen ED, Czujko B, Myhr KM. Pain and sensory complaints in multiple sclerosis. Eur J Neurol. 2004;11(7):479-82.
[53] Weber H, Pfadenhauer K, Stohr M, Rosler A. Central hyperacusis with phonophobia in multiple sclerosis. Mult Scler. 2002;8(6):505-9.
[54] Yamada A, Takeuchi H, Miki H, Touge T, Deguchi K. Acute transverse myelitis associated with ECHO-25 virus infection. Rinsho Shinkeigaku. 1990;30(7):784-6. [Japanese]
[55] Takamura Y, Morimoto S, Tanooka A, Yoshikawa J. Transverse myelitis in a patient with primary antiphospholipid syndrome--a case report. No To Shinkei. 1996;48(9):851-5. [Japanese]
[56] Shian WJ, Chi CS. Acute transverse myelitis in children: clinical analysis of seven cases. Zhonghua Yi Xue Za Zhi (Taipei). 1994;54(1):57-61.
[57] Thomas M, Thomas J, Jr. Acute transverse myelitis. J La State Med Soc. 1997 Feb;149(2):75-7.
[58] Palacio Abizanda FJ, Reina MA, Fornet I, Lopez A, Lopez Lopez MA, Morillas Sendin P. Paresthesia and spinal anesthesia for cesarean section: comparison of patient positioning. Rev Esp Anestesiol Reanim. 2009;56(1):21-6. [Spanish]
[59] Pong RP, Gmelch BS, Bernards CM. Does a paresthesia during spinal needle insertion indicate intrathecal needle placement? Reg Anesth Pain Med. 2009;34(1):29-32.
[60] Fernandez Sdel R, Taboada M, Ulloa B, Rodriguez J, Masid A, Alvarez J. Needle-induced paresthesiae during single-shot spinal anesthesia: a comparison of sitting versus lateral decubitus position. Reg Anesth Pain Med. 2010;35(1):41-4.
[61] Katsuoka H, Watanabe C, Mimori Y, Nakamura S. [A case of vitamin B12 deficiency with broad neurologic disorders and canities]. No To Shinkei. 1997 Mar;49(3):283-6.
[62] Maamar M, Tazi-Mezalek Z, Harmouche H, Ammouri W, Zahlane M, Adnaoui M, et al. Neurological manifestations of vitamin B12 deficiency: a retrospective study of 26 cases. Rev Med Interne. 2006;27(6):442-7. [French]

[63] Juangbhanit C, Nitidanhaprabhas P, Sirimachan S, Areekul S, Tanphaichitr VS. Vitamin B12 deficiency: report of a childhood case. J Med Assoc Thai. 1991;74(6):348-54.
[64] Chan RC, Paine KW, Varughese G. Ulnar neuropathy at the elbow: comparison of simple decompression and anterior transposition. Neurosurgery. 1980;7(6):545-50.
[65] Foti C, Romita P, Vestita M. Unusual presentation of carpal tunnel syndrome with cutaneous signs: a case report and review of the literature. Immunopharmacol Immunotoxicol. 2011.
[66] Gautschi OP, Land M, Hoederath P, Fournier JY, Hildebrandt G, Cadosch D. Carpal tunnel syndrome--modern diagnostic and management. Praxis (Bern 1994). 2010;99(3):163-73. [German]
[67] Chow CS, Hung LK, Chiu CP, Lai KL, Lam LN, Ng ML, et al. Is symptomatology useful in distinguishing between carpal tunnel syndrome and cervical spondylosis? Hand Surg. 2005;10(1):1-5.
[68] Kim JE, Lee SG, Kim EJ, Min BW, Ban JS, Lee JH. Ultrasound-guided Lateral Femoral Cutaneous Nerve Block in Meralgia Paresthetica. Korean J Pain. 2011;24(2):115-8.
[69] Patijn J, Mekhail N, Hayek S, Lataster A, van Kleef M, Van Zundert J. Meralgia Paresthetica. Pain Pract. 2011;11(3):302-8.
[70] Van Veer H, Coosemans W, Pirenne J, Monbaliu D. Acute femoral neuropathy: a rare complication after renal transplantation. Transplant Proc. 2010;42(10):4384-8.
[71] Mondelli M, Giannini F, Reale F. Clinical and electrophysiological findings and follow-up in tarsal tunnel syndrome. Electroencephalogr Clin Neurophysiol. 1998;109(5):418-25.
[72] Kim E, Childers MK. Tarsal tunnel syndrome associated with a pulsating artery: effectiveness of high-resolution ultrasound in diagnosing tarsal tunnel syndrome. J Am Podiatr Med Assoc. 2010;100(3):209-12.
[73] Grovle L, Haugen AJ, Keller A, Natvig B, Brox JI, Grotle M. The bothersomeness of sciatica: patients' self-report of paresthesia, weakness and leg pain. Eur Spine J. 2010;19(2):263-9.
[74] Sharif-Alhoseini M, Rahimi-Movaghar V. Surgical treatment of discogenic sciatica. Neurosciences (Riyadh). 2011;16(1):10-7.
[75] Rahimi-Movaghar V, Rasouli MR, Sharif-Alhoseini M, Jazayeri SB, Vaccaro AR. Discogenic Sciatica: Epidemiology, Etiology, Diagnosis, and Management In: Fonseca D, Martins J, editors. The Sciatic Nerve: Blocks, Injuries and Regeneration. New York: Nova Publishers; 2011.
[76] Herzog J. Use of cervical spine manipulation under anesthesia for management of cervical disk herniation, cervical radiculopathy, and associated cervicogenic headache syndrome. J Manipulative Physiol Ther. 1999;22(3):166-70.
[77] Trummer M, Flaschka G, Unger F, Eustacchio S. Lumbar disc herniation mimicking meralgia paresthetica: case report. Surg Neurol. 2000;54(1):80-1.
[78] Praharaj SS, Vasudev MK, Kolluri VR. Laminoplasty: an evaluation of 24 cases. Neurol India. 2000;48(3):249-54.
[79] Raghavendra S, Vibhin V, Anand HK. F-waves in acute sciatic pressure palsy. Ann Indian Acad Neurol. 2008;11(3):197-8.
[80] Beydoun SR, Sykes SN, Ganguly G, Lee TS. Hereditary neuropathy with liability to pressure palsies: description of seven patients without known family history. Acta Neurologica Scandinavica. 2008;117(4):266-72.

[81] Gyorgy I, Biro A, Mechler F, Molnar MJ. Hereditary neuropathy with liability to pressure palsy in childhood. Ideggyogy Sz. 2008;61(11-12):423-5.
[82] Kumar N, Muley S, Pakiam A, Parry GJ. Phenotypic Variability Leads to Under-recognition of HNPP. Journal of Clinical Neuromuscular Disease. 2002;3(3):106-12.
[83] Bird TD. Charcot-Marie-Tooth Hereditary Neuropathy Overview. 1993.
[84] Mazzeo A, Muglia M, Rodolico C, Toscano A, Patitucci A, Quattrone A, et al. Charcot-Marie-Tooth disease type 1B: marked phenotypic variation of the Ser78Leu mutation in five Italian families. Acta Neurol Scand. 2008;118(5):328-32.
[85] Kyle RA, Bayrd ED. Amyloidosis: review of 236 cases. Medicine (Baltimore). 1975;54(4):271-99.
[86] Price CJS, Evangelou N, Gregory R. Amyloid neuropathy presenting as thoraco-abdominal parathesia. European Journal of Neurology. 2002;9(2):185-.
[87] Novak CB, Mackinnon SE. Nerve injury in repetitive motion disorders. Clin Orthop Relat Res. 1998;(351):10-20.
[88] Woolf CJ, Mannion RJ. Neuropathic pain: aetiology, symptoms, mechanisms, and management. Lancet. 1999;353(9168):1959-64.
[89] Landi L, Manicone PF, Piccinelli S, Raia A, Raia R. A novel surgical approach to impacted mandibular third molars to reduce the risk of paresthesia: a case series. J Oral Maxillofac Surg. 2010;68(5):969-74.
[90] Bataineh AB. Sensory nerve impairment following mandibular third molar surgery. J Oral Maxillofac Surg. 2001;59(9):1012-7.
[91] Sanders RJ, Hammond SL, Rao NM. Diagnosis of thoracic outlet syndrome. J Vasc Surg. 2007;46(3):601-4.
[92] Kempler P. Clinical presentation and diagnosis of diabetic neuropathy. Orv Hetil. 2002;143(20):1113-20. [Hungarian]
[93] Koike H, Sobue G. Alcoholic neuropathy. Curr Opin Neurol. 2006;19(5):481-6.
[94] Schuchardt V. Alcohol and the peripheral nervous system. Ther Umsch. 2000;57(4):196-9. [German]
[95] Schutt M, Lorch H, Kruger S, Klingenberg RD, Peters A, Klein HH. Recurrent hypoglycemia caused by malignant insulinoma: chemoembolization as a therapeutic option. Med Klin (Munich). 2001;96(10):632-6. [German]
[96] Blum JA, Schmid C, Hatz C, Kazumba L, Mangoni P, Rutishauser J, et al. Sleeping glands? - The role of endocrine disorders in sleeping sickness (T.b. gambiense Human African Trypanosomiasis). Acta Trop. 2007;104(1):16-24.
[97] Djrolo F, Houngbe F, Attolou V, Hountondji B, Quenum K, Hountondji A. Hypothyroidism: clinical and etiological aspects in Cotonou (Republic of Benin). Sante. 2001;11(4):245-9. [French]
[98] Duyff RF, Van den Bosch J, Laman DM, van Loon BJ, Linssen WH. Neuromuscular findings in thyroid dysfunction: a prospective clinical and electrodiagnostic study. J Neurol Neurosurg Psychiatry. 2000;68(6):750-5.
[99] Maeda SS, Fortes EM, Oliveira UM, Borba VC, Lazaretti-Castro M. Hypoparathyroidism and pseudohypoparathyroidism. Arq Bras Endocrinol Metabol. 2006;50(4):664-73.
[100] Skugor M. Hypocalcemia. 2011; http://www.clevelandclinicmeded.com [cited 2011 June 12]
[101] anonymous. Adernal gland. Professional guide to diseases. 9 ed. Pennsylvania: Lippincott Williams & Wilkins; 2008. p. 628-42.

[102] Shakhatreh FM, Mas'ad D. Menopausal symptoms and health problems of women aged 50-65 years in southern Jordan. Climacteric. 2006;9(4):305-11.
[103] Bensaleh H, Belgnaoui FZ, Douira L, Berbiche L, Senouci K, Hassam B. Skin and menopause. Ann Endocrinol (Paris). 2006;67(6):575-80. [French]
[104] Moriwaki K, Kanno Y, Nakamoto H, Okada H, Suzuki H. Vitamin B6 deficiency in elderly patients on chronic peritoneal dialysis. Adv Perit Dial. 2000;16:308-12.
[105] Ondo WG. Restless legs syndrome. Neurol Clin. 2005;23(4):1165-85, viii.
[106] Mehta M, Rath GP, Padhy UP, Marda M, Mahajan C, Dash HH. Intensive care management of patients with acute intermittent porphyria: Clinical report of four cases and review of literature. Indian J Crit Care Med. 2010;14(2):88-91.
[107] Sugimura K. Acute intermittent porphyria. Nippon Rinsho. 1995;53(6):1418-21. [Japanese]
[108] Blondeau JM, Aoki FY, Galvin GB, Nagy JI. Characterization of acute and latent herpes simplex virus infection of dorsal root ganglia in rats. Lab Anim. 1991;25(2):97-105.
[109] Shiraki K, Andoh T, Imakita M, Kurokawa M, Kuraishi Y, Niimura M, et al. Caffeine inhibits paresthesia induced by herpes simplex virus through action on primary sensory neurons in rats. Neurosci Res. 1998;31(3):235-40.
[110] Juntas Morales R, Tillier JN, Davous P. Facial diplegia and acute inflammatory demyelinating neuropathy secondary to varicella. Rev Neurol (Paris). 2009;165(10):836-8. [French]
[111] Takei-Suzuki M, Hayashi Y, Kimura A, Nagasawa M, Koumura A, Sakurai T, et al. Case of varicella myelitis in nursing care worker. Brain Nerve. 2008;60(1):79-83. [Japanese]
[112] Gross G, Schofer H, Wassilew S, Friese K, Timm A, Guthoff R, et al. Herpes zoster guideline of the German Dermatology Society (DDG). J Clin Virol. 2003;26(3):277-89; discussion 91-3.
[113] Carbone V, Leonardi A, Pavese M, Raviola E, Giordano M. Herpes zoster of the trigeminal nerve: a case report and review of the literature. Minerva Stomatol. 2004;53(1-2):49-59. [Italian]
[114] anonymous. Shingles Symptoms Information. 2008; http://shinglessymptomsguide.com [cited 2011 June 20]
[115] Pasqualucci A. Herpes Zoster and post-herpetic neuralgia: everything to revise?. Minerva Anestesiol. 1999;65(7-8):541-8. [Italian]
[116] Goh CL, Khoo L. A retrospective study of the clinical presentation and outcome of herpes zoster in a tertiary dermatology outpatient referral clinic. Int J Dermatol. 1997;36(9):667-72.
[117] Boskey E. What is the Difference Between Cold Sores, Canker Sores, & Chancre? 2009; http://std.about.com [cited 2011 June 25]
[118] Santhosh K, Surbhi L, Harish T, Jyothi T, Arvind T, Prabu D, et al. Do active ingredients in non alcoholic chlorhexidine mouth wash provide added effectiveness? Observations from a randomized controlled trial. Odontostomatol Trop. 2010;33(130):26-34.
[119] Logigian EL, Kaplan RF, Steere AC. Chronic neurologic manifestations of Lyme disease. N Engl J Med. 1990;323(21):1438-44.
[120] Logigian EL, Steere AC. Clinical and electrophysiologic findings in chronic neuropathy of Lyme disease. Neurology. 1992;42(2):303-11.

[121] Verma A. Epidemiology and clinical features of HIV-1 associated neuropathies. J Peripher Nerv Syst. 2001;6(1):8-13.
[122] Araujo AP, Nascimento OJ, Garcia OS. Distal sensory polyneuropathy in a cohort of HIV-infected children over five years of age. Pediatrics. 2000;106(3):E35.
[123] Ramos-e-Silva M, Rebello PF. Leprosy. Recognition and treatment. Am J Clin Dermatol. 2001;2(4):203-11.
[124] Kumar B, Kaur I, Dogra S, Kumaran MS. Pure neuritic leprosy in India: an appraisal. Int J Lepr Other Mycobact Dis. 2004;72(3):284-90.
[125] Pavlovic DM, Milovic AM. Clinical characteristics and therapy of neurosyphilis in patients who are negative for human immunodeficiency virus. Srp Arh Celok Lek. 1999;127(7-8):236-40. [Serbian]
[126] Berger JR. Spinal cord syphilis associated with human immunodeficiency virus infection: a treatable myelopathy. Am J Med. 1992;92(1):101-3.
[127] Matijosaitis V, Vaitkus A, Pauza V, Valiukeviciene S, Gleizniene R. Neurosyphilis manifesting as spinal transverse myelitis. Medicina (Kaunas). 2006;42(5):401-5.
[128] Viegas GV. Guillain-Barre syndrome. Review and presentation of a case with pedal manifestations. J Am Podiatr Med Assoc. 1997;87(5):209-18.
[129] Shian WJ, Chi CS. Guillain-Barre syndrome in infants and children. Zhonghua Yi Xue Za Zhi (Taipei). 1994 Aug;54(2):131-5.
[130] Mattner F, Henke-Gendo C, Martens A, Drosten C, Schulz TF, Heim A, et al. Risk of rabies infection and adverse effects of postexposure prophylaxis in healthcare workers and other patient contacts exposed to a rabies virus-infected lung transplant recipient. Infect Control Hosp Epidemiol. 2007;28(5):513-8.
[131] Koruk ST, Un H, Gursoy B, Unal N, Calisir C, Unutmaz G, et al. A human rabies case with antemortem diagnosis. Mikrobiyol Bul. 2010;44(2):303-9. [Turkish]
[132] Kumar V, Fausto N, Abbas A. Robbins and Cotran Pathologic Basis of Disease Philadelphia: Elsevier/Saunders; 2004.
[133] Chiardola F, Schneeberger EE, Citera G, Rosemffet GM, Kuo L, Santillan G, et al. Prevalence and clinical significance of eosinophilia in patients with rheumatoid arthritis in Argentina. J Clin Rheumatol. 2008;14(4):211-3.
[134] Falope ZF, Griffiths ID, Platt PN, Todd NV. Cervical myelopathy and rheumatoid arthritis: a retrospective analysis of management. Clin Rehabil. 2002;16(6):625-9.
[135] Grant IA, Hunder GG, Homburger HA, Dyck PJ. Peripheral neuropathy associated with sicca complex. Neurology. 1997;48(4):855-62.
[136] Mellgren SI, Goransson LG, Omdal R. Primary Sjogren's syndrome associated neuropathy. Can J Neurol Sci. 2007;34(3):280-7.
[137] Olsen ML, Arnett FC, Rosenbaum D, Grotta J, Warner NB. Sjogren's syndrome and other rheumatic disorders presenting to a neurology service. J Autoimmun. 1989;2(4):477-83.
[138] Reichel H, Liebhaber A, Babinsky K, Keysser G. [Radiological changes in the cervical spine in rheumatoid arthritis -- prognostic factors obtained by a cross-sectional study]. Z Rheumatol. 2002;61(6):710-7.
[139] Gisondi P, Girolomoni G, Sampogna F, Tabolli S, Abeni D. Prevalence of psoriatic arthritis and joint complaints in a large population of Italian patients hospitalised for psoriasis. Eur J Dermatol. 2005;15(4):279-83.
[140] Bruckle W, Zeidler H. Fibromyalgia. Internist (Berl). 2004;45(8):923-32; quiz 33-4. [German]

[141] Cacace E, Ruggiero V, Anedda C, Denotti A, Minerba L, Perpignano G. Quality of life and associated clinical distress in fibromyalgia. Reumatismo. 2006;58(3):226-9. [Italian]
[142] Rolfe M, Beri-beri. Endemic amongst urban Gambians. Afr Health. 1994;16(3):22-3.
[143] Lasinski T. Sensory polyneuropathy caused by pantothenic acid deficiency. Wiad Lek. 1978;31(17):1227-9. [Polish]
[144] Veldhuis SK, Witjes MJ, Reintsema H, Roodenburg JL, Schepman KP, Timmenga NM, et al. Cheek paresthesia by an osteosarcoma. Ned Tijdschr Tandheelkd. 2010;117(4):215-8. [Dutch]
[145] Khine AA, Prabhakaran VC, Selva D. Idiopathic sclerosing orbital inflammation: two cases presenting with paresthesia. Ophthal Plast Reconstr Surg. 2009;25(1):65-7.
[146] Huang JS, Ho YP, Ho KY, Wu YM, Chen CC, Wang CC, et al. Multiple myeloma with oral manifestations--report of two cases. Kaohsiung J Med Sci. 1997;13(6):388-94. [Chinese]
[147] Lipponi G, Gasparrini PM, Lucantoni C, Cadeddu G, Gaetti R. Peripheral neuropathy and multiple myeloma in aging: a case report. Arch Gerontol Geriatr. 1992;15 Suppl 1:229-35.
[148] Kim SK, Park IK, Park BH, Park W, Lee HS, Kim TH, et al. A case report: isolated a heavy chain monoclonal gammopathy in a patient with polyneuropathy, organomegaly, endocrinopathy, monoclonal gammopathy and skin change syndrome. Int J Clin Pract Suppl. 2005(147):26-30.
[149] Malenfant A, Forget R, Papillon J, Amsel R, Frigon JY, Choiniere M. Prevalence and characteristics of chronic sensory problems in burn patients. Pain. 1996;67(2-3):493-500.
[150] Choiniere M, Melzack R, Papillon J. Pain and paresthesia in patients with healed burns: an exploratory study. J Pain Symptom Manage. 1991;6(7):437-44.
[151] Tomkins KL, Holland AJ. Electrical burn injuries in children. J Paediatr Child Health. 2008 Nov 28.
[152] Singerman J, Gomez M, Fish JS. Long-term sequelae of low-voltage electrical injury. J Burn Care Res. 2008;29(5):773-7.
[153] Berg A, Aas P, Lund T. Frostbite injuries. Tidsskr Nor Laegeforen. 1999;119(3):382-5. [Norwegian]
[154] Marci M, D'Aleo F, Mignano Maru R, Termini D, Tumminello M. Atrial septal defect in a child with Ito syndrome. Ital Heart J Suppl. 2004;5(3):218-20. [Italian]
[155] Dinehart SM, Dillard R, Raimer SS, Diven S, Cobos R, Pupo R. Cutaneous manifestations of acrodynia (pink disease). Arch Dermatol. 1988;124(1):107-9.
[156] Boyd AS, Seger D, Vannucci S, Langley M, Abraham JL, King LE, Jr. Mercury exposure and cutaneous disease. J Am Acad Dermatol. 2000;43(1 Pt 1):81-90.
[157] Battaglia C, Mancini F, Persico N, Paradisi R, Busacchi P, Venturoli S. Doppler flow analysis of the palmaris superficial branch of the radial artery in postmenopausal women with acroparesthesia: the role of hormone therapy. A pilot study. Climacteric. 2011;14(1):181-4.
[158] Tseng CW, Wu CC, Tsai KC, Chen WJ. Acute paresthesia in a patient with migraine. J Clin Neurosci. 2010;17(11):1474-5.
[159] Monteso Curto MP, Ferre i Grau C, Martinez Quintana V. Fibromyalgia: beyond the depression. Rev Enferm. 2010;33(9):20-6. [Spanish]
[160] Praharaj SK, Arora M. Sertraline-induced facial paresthesia. J Clin Psychopharmacol. 2007;27(6):725.

[161] Ponticelli C, Campise MR. Neurological complications in kidney transplant recipients. J Nephrol. 2005;18(5):521-8.
[162] Poza JJ, Cobo AM, Marti-Masso JF. Neuropathy associated with arteriosclerosis. Rev Neurol. 1997;25(144):1194-7. [Spanish]
[163] Sinczuk-Walczak H, Szymczak M, Halatek T. Effects of occupational exposure to arsenic on the nervous system: clinical and neurophysiological studies. Int J Occup Med Environ Health. 2010;23(4):347-55.
[164] Kuruvilla A, Pillay VV, Adhikari P, Venkatesh T, Chakrapani M, Rao HT, et al. Clinical manifestations of lead workers of Mangalore, India. Toxicol Ind Health. 2006;22(9):405-13.
[165] Marie RM, Le Biez E, Busson P, Schaeffer S, Boiteau L, Dupuy B, et al. Nitrous oxide anesthesia-associated myelopathy. Arch Neurol. 2000;57(3):380-2.
[166] Lin CY, Guo WY, Chen SP, Chen JT, Kao KP, Wu ZA, et al. Neurotoxicity of nitrous oxide: multimodal evoked potentials in an abuser. Clin Toxicol (Phila). 2007;45(1):67-71.
[167] Roth D, Hubmann N, Havel C, Herkner H, Schreiber W, Laggner A. Victim of carbon monoxide poisoning identified by carbon monoxide oximetry. J Emerg Med. 2011;40(6):640-2.
[168] Gold BS, Dart RC, Barish RA. Bites of venomous snakes. N Engl J Med. 2002;347(5):347-56.
[169] Derouiche F, Cohen E, Rodier G, Boulay C, Courtois S. Ciguatera and peripheral neuropathy: a case report. Rev Neurol (Paris). 2000;156(5):514-6. [French]
[170] Arcila-Herrera H, Castello-Navarrete A, Mendoza-Ayora J, Montero-Cervantes L, Gonzalez-Franco MF, Brito-Villanueva WO. Ten cases of Ciguatera fish poisoning in Yucatan. Rev Invest Clin. 1998;50(2):149-52. [Spanish]
[171] Grau C. Damage to the spinal medulla caused by radiation. Ugeskr Laeger. 1993;155(4):208-11. [Danish]
[172] Marshall R, Gupta ND, Palacios E, Neitzschman HR. Progressive paresthesia and weakness after intrathecal chemotherapy. J La State Med Soc. 2008;160(2):92-4.
[173] Lucke T, Hoppner W, Schmidt E, Illsinger S, Das AM. Fabry disease: reduced activities of respiratory chain enzymes with decreased levels of energy-rich phosphates in fibroblasts. Mol Genet Metab. 2004;82(1):93-7.
[174] Strujic BJ, Jeren T. Fabry disease--a diagnostic and therapeutic problem. Ren Fail. 2005;27(6):783-6.
[175] Wierzbicki AS, Lloyd MD, Schofield CJ, Feher MD, Gibberd FB. Refsum's disease: a peroxisomal disorder affecting phytanic acid alpha-oxidation. J Neurochem. 2002;80(5):727-35.
[176] Gatti RA. Ataxia-telangiectasia. Dermatol Clin. 1995;13(1):1-6.
[177] Chun HH, Gatti RA. Ataxia-telangiectasia, an evolving phenotype. DNA Repair (Amst). 2004;3(8-9):1187-96.
[178] Feki I, Belahsen F, Ben Jemaa M, Mhiri C. Subacute myelitis revealed by human immunodeficiency virus infection. Rev Neurol (Paris). 2003;159(5 Pt 1):577-80. [French]